RHYTHM

The Cellular Mode of Communication

THE BOOK ON VIBRATION SCIENCE

PROF DR SYED MOHAMMAD WARIS

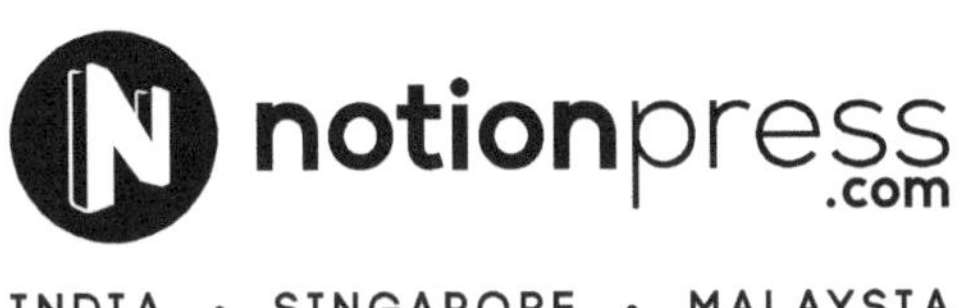

INDIA • SINGAPORE • MALAYSIA

ISBN
Paperback 979-8-89632-789-9
Hardcase 979-8-89673-380-5

Rhythm

The cellular Mode Of Communication

The book on vibration Science

(for Medical Students and Practitioners)

Author

Prof Syed Mohammad Waris Ph.D.

Associate Academic Director at London academy of Sports and Health science UK

Professor at MPR International school Switzerland

CONTENTS

PREFACE

Dear Doctors, Greetings, This book will introduce to you a new concept of we as Vibrational beings.

This book will connect you with the vibrational science. Along with the Concept of wave particle dualism. The endless human connection beyond the solar system and how we are connected to earth, universe and to each other.

This Book of vibration science is to link recent scientific advances of vibration as therapy.

This book is dedicated to all the Medical students and practitioners

This Book will be as a text book for my upcoming workshops and fellowship programs

I have tried to make this book error free but sincerely apologize for any mistake that may have escaped my notice.

I will highly appreciate the suggestions and criticism are most welcome from readers for the improvement of this book.

With Best Regards

Prof. Syed Mohammad Waris

PhD (Vibration Science).

BPT (RGUHS, India), MSC Physical therapy (US),

FNR (LASHS, UK), CYT.

MIAP, MIRS, FRHS, AMPLR(UK), MSJA(Malaysia), MWSO(Switzerland).

Certified Matrix rhythm practitioner (Germany)

Certified Pro Vib practitioner (Austria).

Associate director academics at London academy of sports and health sciences UK

Professor at MPR Science School Switzerland

1

WAVE–PARTICLE DUALITY

Louis Victor Pierre Raymond, 7th Duc de Broglie (15 August 1892 – 19 March 1987) was a French physicist and aristocrat who made groundbreaking contributions to quantum theory. In his 1924 PhD thesis, he postulated the wave nature of electrons and suggested that all matter has wave properties. This concept is known as the de Broglie hypothesis, an example of wave–particle duality, and forms a central part of the theory of quantum mechanics.

De Broglie won the Nobel Prize for Physics in 1929, after the wave-like behavior of matter was first experimentally demonstrated in 1927.

The 1925 pilot-wave model, and the wave-like behavior of particles discovered by de Broglie was used by Erwin Schrödinger in his formulation of wave mechanics. The pilot-wave model and interpretation was then abandoned, in favor of the quantum formalism, until 1952 when it was rediscovered and enhanced by David Bohm.

MATTER AND WAVE–PARTICLE DUALITY

Main article: De Broglie hypothesis

Studying the nature of X-ray radiation and discussing its properties with his brother Maurice, who considered these rays to be some kind of combination of waves and particles, contributed to Louis de Broglie's awareness of the need to build a theory linking particle and wave representations. In addition, he was familiar with the works (1919–1922) of Marcel Brillouin, which proposed a hydrodynamic model of an atom and attempted to relate it to the results of Bohr's theory. The starting point in the work of Louis de Broglie was the idea of A. Einstein about the quanta of light. In his first article on this subject, published in 1922, the French scientist considered blackbody radiation as a gas of light quanta and, using classical statistical mechanics, derived the Wien radiation law in the framework of such a representation. In his next publication, he tried to reconcile the concept of light quanta with the phenomena of interference and diffraction and came to the conclusion that it was necessary to associate a certain periodicity with quanta. In this case, light quanta were interpreted by him as relativistic particles of very small mass.

It remained to extend the wave considerations to any massive particles, and in the summer of 1923 a decisive breakthrough occurred. De Broglie outlined his ideas in a short note "Waves and quanta" (French: Ondes et quanta, presented at a meeting of the Paris Academy of Sciences on September 10, 1923),which marked the beginning of the creation of wave mechanics. In this paper and his subsequent PhD thesis,the scientist suggested that a moving particle with energy E and velocity v is characterized by some internal periodic process with a frequency E/h (later known as Compton frequency), where h is Planck's constant. To reconcile these considerations, based on the quantum principle, with the ideas of special relativity, de Broglie associated wave he called a “phase wave” with a moving body, which propagates with the phase velocity c2/v. Such a wave, which later received the name matter wave, or de Broglie wave, in the process of body movement remains in phase with the internal periodic process. Having then examined the motion of an electron in a closed orbit, the scientist showed that the requirement for phase matching directly leads to the quantum Bohr-Sommerfeld condition, that is, to quantize the angular momentum. In the next two notes (reported at the meetings on September 24 and October 8, respectively), de Broglie came to the conclusion that the particle velocity is equal to the group velocity of phase waves, and the particle moves along the normal to surfaces of equal phase. In the general case, the trajectory of a particle can be determined using Fermat’s principle (for waves) or the principle of least action (for particles), which indicates a connection between geometric optics and classical mechanics.

This theory set the basis of wave mechanics. It was supported by Einstein, confirmed by the electron diffraction experiments of G P Thomson and Davisson and Germer, and generalized by the work of Schrödinger.

From a philosophical viewpoint, this theory of matter-waves has contributed greatly to the ruin of the atomism of the past. Originally, de Broglie thought that real wave (i.e., having a direct physical interpretation) was associated with particles. In fact, the wave aspect of matter was formalized by a wavefunction defined by the Schrödinger equation, which is a pure mathematical entity having a probabilistic interpretation, without the support of real physical elements. This wavefunction gives an appearance of wave behavior to matter, without making real physical waves appear. However, until the end of his life de Broglie returned to a direct and real physical interpretation of matter-waves, following the work of David Bohm.

CONJECTURE OF AN INTERNAL CLOCK OF THE ELECTRON

In his 1924 thesis, de Broglie conjectured that the electron has an internal clock that constitutes part of the mechanism by which a pilot wave guides a particle.Subsequently, David Hestenes has proposed a link to the zitterbewegung that was suggested by Erwin Schrödinger.

While attempts at verifying the internal clock hypothesis and measuring clock frequency are so far not conclusive, recent experimental data is at least compatible with de Broglie's conjecture.

NON-NULLITY AND VARIABILITY OF MASS

According to de Broglie, the neutrino and the photon have rest masses that are non-zero, though very low. That a photon is not quite massless is imposed by the coherence of his theory. Incidentally, this rejection of the hypothesis of a massless photon enabled him to doubt the hypothesis of the expansion of the universe.

In addition, he believed that the true mass of particles is not constant, but variable, and that each particle can be represented as a thermodynamic machine equivalent to a cyclic integral of action.

GENERALIZATION OF THE PRINCIPLE OF LEAST ACTION

In the second part of his 1924 thesis, de Broglie used the equivalence of the mechanical principle of least action with Fermat's optical principle: "Fermat's principle applied to phase waves is identical to Maupertuis' principle applied to the moving body; the possible dynamic trajectories of the moving body are identical to the possible rays of the wave." This equivalence had been pointed out by Hamilton a century earlier, and published by him around 1830, in an era where no experience gave proof of the fundamental principles of physics being involved in the description of atomic phenomena.

Up to his final work, he appeared to be the physicist who most sought that dimension of action which Max Planck, at the beginning of the 20th century, had shown to be the only universal unity (with his dimension of entropy).

DUALITY OF THE LAWS OF NATURE

Far from claiming to make "the contradiction disappear" which Max Born thought could be achieved with a statistical approach, de Broglie extended wave–particle duality to all particles (and to crystals which revealed the effects of diffraction) and extended the principle of duality to the laws of nature.

His last work made a single system of laws from the two large systems of thermodynamics and of mechanics:

When Boltzmann and his continuators developed their statistical interpretation of Thermodynamics, one could have considered Thermodynamics to be a complicated branch of Dynamics. But, with my actual ideas, it's Dynamics that appear to be a simplified branch of Thermodynamics. I think that, of all the ideas that I've introduced in quantum theory in these past years, it's that idea that is, by far, the most important and the most profound.

That idea seems to match the continuous–discontinuous duality, since its dynamics could be the limit of its thermodynamics when transitions to continuous limits are postulated. It is also close to that of Leibniz, who posited the necessity of "architectonic principles" to complete the system of mechanical laws.

However, according to him, there is less duality, in the sense of opposition, than synthesis (one is the limit of the other) and the effort of synthesis is constant according to him, like in his first formula, in which the first member pertains to mechanics and the second to optics:

$$mc^2 = h\nu$$

NEUTRINO THEORY OF LIGHT

Main article: Neutrino theory of light

This theory, which dates from 1934, introduces the idea that the photon is equivalent to the fusion of two Dirac neutrinos. It is not currently accepted by the majority of physicists.

HIDDEN THERMODYNAMICS

De Broglie's final idea was the hidden thermodynamics of isolated particles. It is an attempt to bring together the three furthest principles of physics: the principles of Fermat, Maupertuis, and Carnot.

In this work, action becomes a sort of opposite to entropy, through an equation that relates the only two universal dimensions of the form:

$$\frac{\text{action}}{h} = -\frac{\text{entropy}}{k}$$

As a consequence of its great impact, this theory brings back the uncertainty principle to distances around extrema of action, distances corresponding to reductions in entropy.

2

CONNECTIVITY

We all are vibrational beings. As we now know about the wave particle dualism (matter has both wave and particle nature) applies on us as well.

Healthy muscles vibrate in the frequency range of 8 to 12 Hz. This can be observed directly on the cellular level. Muscle cells pulsate, Any Change in the rhythm of pulsation detected with the help of piezoelectric sensors outside the normal range correlate positively with Pain, muscle tension and other health problem. Changed muscle elasticity and plasticity are also linked to the change in the frequency and in the logistics of the living process on the cellular level.

THE ENDLESS HUMAN CONNECTION BEYOND THE SOLAR SYSTEM

"We are all connected; To each other, biologically. To the earth, chemically. To the rest of the universe atomically."

—Neil DeGrasse Tyson

Human body within is connected cell ...tissue....organ...organ system

Our connection to the Earth – to Nature – is one of the most important connections humans have.

Without Nature, without the Earth, we would not exist. Our human bodies are connected to the Earth, the Solar System, and beyond.

Whatever happens to the Earth happens to us. If the planet heats up, we heat up.

When the Earth changes its axis position, we change our axis position. We have long forgotten that the magnetic field inside our bodies lines up with the Earth's magnetic field, and when the Earth's magnetism shifts, we physically shift with it.

In the same way, the massive and diverse Universe, with its trillions of galaxies and solar systems, influences everything in the same way to assure stability and balance

All the planets in our Solar System are in constant motion. Like the human body, all planets resonate, they circulate heat, and they move around a central sun.

Like humans, the Solar System produces energy, it circulates heat, and it moves around a central Galaxy.

Just like us, the Galaxy resonates, it circulates heat, and it moves around a central Universal core.

We are all connected. We all move together in a fine-tuned and very precise symphony.

The next time you feel isolated, different, or possibly "superior" to any other form of life, think about this connection. Humans are but a small piece of a massive creation.

We are all connected. We all move together in a fine-tuned and very precise symphony.

The next time you feel isolated, different, or possibly "superior" to any other form of life, think about this connection. Humans are but a small piece of a massive creation.

3

CONCEPT OF VIBRATION THERAPY

VIBRATION SCIENCE

Whole Body Vibration Therapy

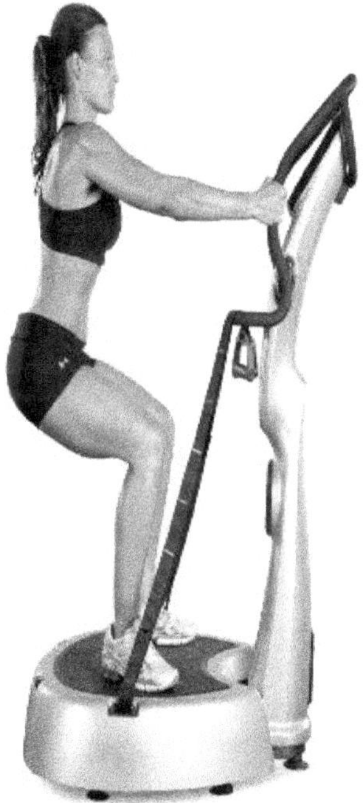

Fig 2.4 *Basic position on whole body vibration platform*

Vibration platform for the whole body.

The idea originated in space science: **B**io**M**echanical **S**timulation (BMS) by means of whole-body vibration.

In 1856, Russain physican and inventor Gustav Zander developed a series of machines that utilized weights and pulleys to create a sense of vibration. The purpose of apparatus was therapeutic.

In 1895, Dr. Jhon Harvey Kellogg implemented vibration therapy in his health practice.

With a vibration chair he developed himself, he claimed the therapy was good for circulation and could also alleviate constipation.

During the Russian space program, Physicians noticed that the returning astronauts suffered from loss of bone mass & bone fractures at a much earlier age than was normal.

They began to use whole body vibration device to help strengthen astronaut's bone mass & muscles.

Today NASA uses VT to help prevent muscle loss in astronauts.

HOW DOES VIBRATION THERAPY WORK?

4

WHOLE BODY VIBRATION

During whole-body vibration therapy, your therapist will ask you to stand, sit, or lay on a machine supported by a vibrating platform. For example, they may ask you to stand in a half-squat position with your knees bent.

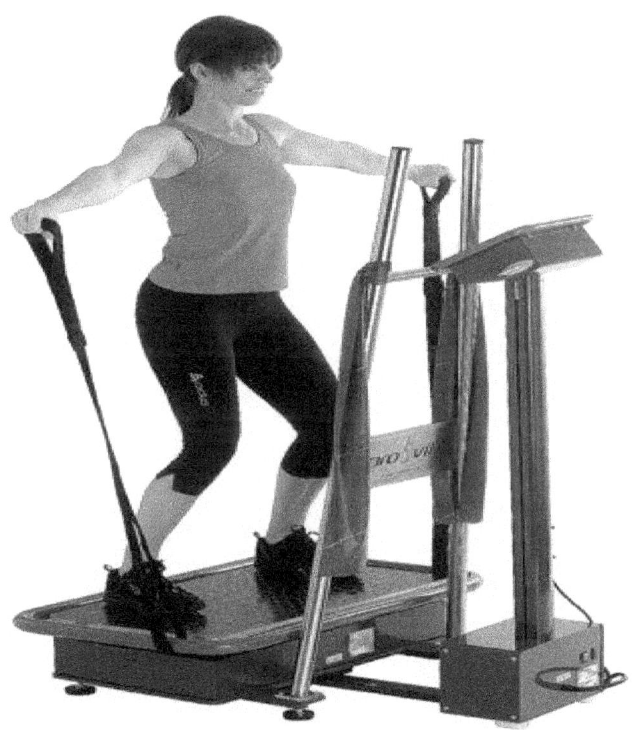

Fig 2.5 *Balance training on vibration platform*

5

TYPES OF WHOLD-BODY VIBRATION MACHINES

1. PIVOTAL

In Pivotal vibration machines, the platform you stand on tilts around a central pivot point like a see-saw. The left and right sides alternate up and down while the centre remains fixed.

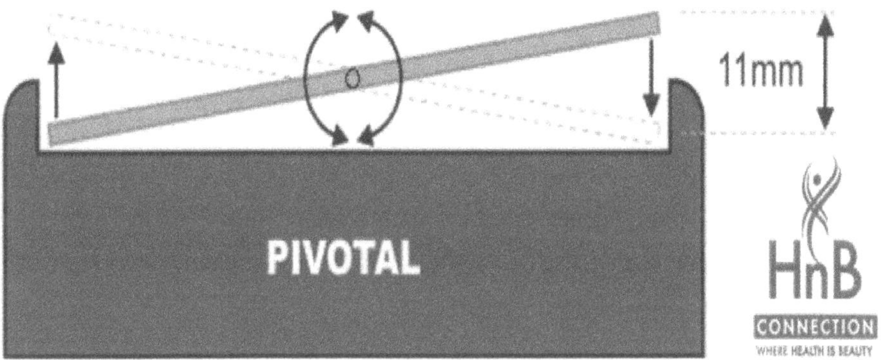

Fig 2.6 *Pivotal vibration machine*

2. LINEAL

In an attempt to compete with the successful German vibration platforms, a Dutch company created a vibration machine with a new kind of platform movement called Lineal.

A Lineal vibration platform remains horizontal at all times with the entire platform moving up and down by the same amount.

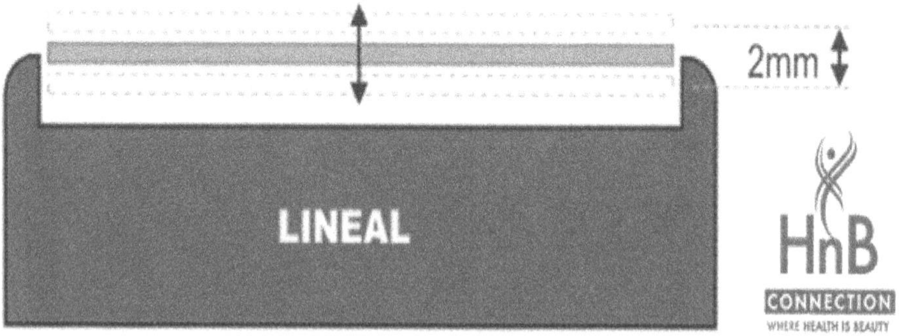

Fig 2.7 *Lineal vibration machine*

VERTICAL VIBRATION (TRI-PLANAR, VERTICAL UNIFORM, STRAIGHT)

How does the platform move? The platform moves straight up and down. Vertical vibration units tend to have platform motion with lower amplitude (about 2 – 4 mm) and often achieve comfortable frequencies (between 20 – 50 Hz).

Vertical vibration

What happens inside the body? The vibration stimulus travels straight up through the body. The user's whole body weight is being mobilized; lymphatic fluids are being circulated well.

Who is this best for? This is typically the best type of vibration for stronger and more active users. It is excellent for accelerated fitness training along with building and toning muscle. It is also a great help for combating Osteoporosis because it maximizes lymph drainage and promotes the release of osteoblast.

How DC's apply vertical vibration: DC's use vertical vibration to enhance muscle building and proprioceptive response in rehabilitation regiments once the patient is out of the acute phase. Many DC's use vertical vibration to treat osteoporosis because a weight bearing load **is** placed on the patient's entire skeletal structure. This type of WBV is also fantastic for lymph drainage and can be used for a pre-adjustment warm up.

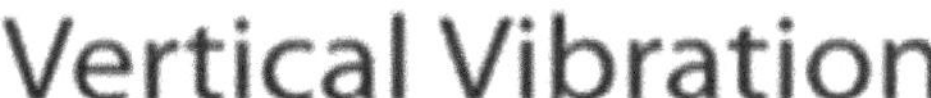

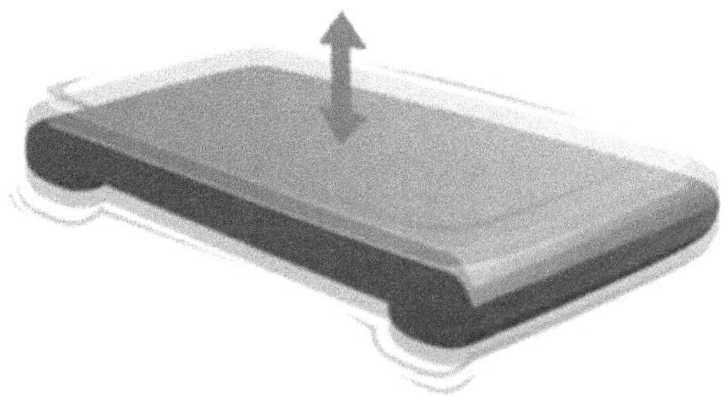

OSCILLATING VIBRATION (TRIANGULAR OSCILLATING, VERTICAL ALTERNATE VIBRATION, PIVOTAL, TOGGLE)

How does the platform move? The motor drives a toggle mechanism that elevates one side of the platform, then the other side, sometimes described as a "teeter-totter" motion. Comparatively, Oscillating units have higher amplitude (up to 10 mm or 1 cm) and lower frequency (5 – 35 Hz).

Oscillating vibration

What happens inside the body? Slow motion filming of the thigh, hip and abdominal areas show the incredible wave motion of subcutaneous fat, lending credence to the weight-loss/trimming ability of this modality. It contributes greatly to mobilization and activates the core muscles. Also great for increasing the metabolism and burning calories which aids in weight loss!

Who is this best for? It's great for patients who suffer from lack of mobility in the lumbar and sacroiliac areas, core muscle weakness or generally have not exercised or been mobile for quite some time. It is the perfect type of vibration for the baby boomer and not-so athletic user who is interested in getting started and wants to feel better quickly.

How DC's apply oscillating vibration: DC's use oscillating vibration equipment for patients who are stiff, lack core strength, and want to get their bodies stimulated, start exercising, and get moving. As society in the United States becomes more aware and conscious about healthy living, DC's have been using oscillating units in conjunction with weight-loss initiatives in their practice.

Oscillating Vibration

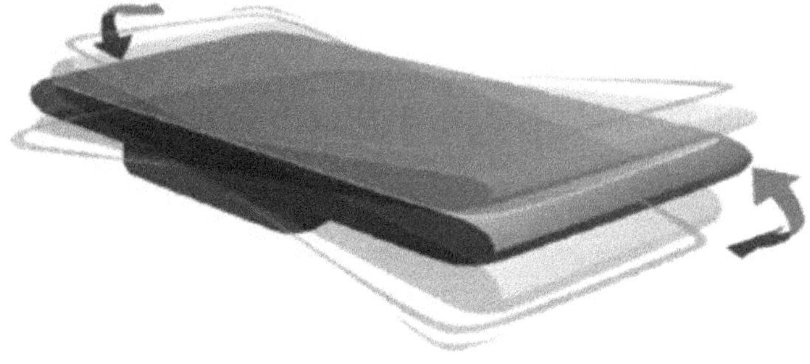

ELLIPTICAL VIBRATION (LOW-INTENSITY VERTICAL, 3-DIMENSIONAL)

How does the platform move? In these units, the motion is created by a vertically placed motor that has uneven centrifugal plates attached to it. This produces an elliptical motion of the platform which is the mildest form of vibration out of the three types. PowerVibe often compares Elliptical vibration to be a low intensity form of Vertical vibration. Comparatively, Elliptical units have lower amplitude (2 – 4 mm) and often function at higher frequency (20 – 50 Hz).

What happens inside the body? this is the most benign form of vibration that lends itself likely to be the best modality to stimulate the proprioceptive system. This is our innate balance system, which helps our body to orient itself in the 3 dimensional world. It stabilizes the body and gives us our sense of equilibrium.ellipticalvibration

Who is this best for? Elliptical Vibration works great for elderly users with balance issues and circulation problems and those who just want to increase their daily activities. Many of these users have been sedentary for a number of years and are not comfortable with the intensity of vertical or oscillating units. This is also the preferred type of unit for stroke patients or other central nervous system (CNS) issues. It is the perfect type of WBV for seniors or users under 150 lbs body weight!

How DC's apply vertical vibration: In the practice, DC's have had great success using elliptical vibration units to enhance rehabilitation plans even when the patient is in the acute phase of an injury. Unilateral exercises can be performed to focus on a specific part of the body and the vibration stimulus accelerates rehabilitation at a phenomenal rate. DC's find that elliptical units are also fantastic for drastically improving proprioception, balance, and stability for geriatric patients.

Elliptical Vibration

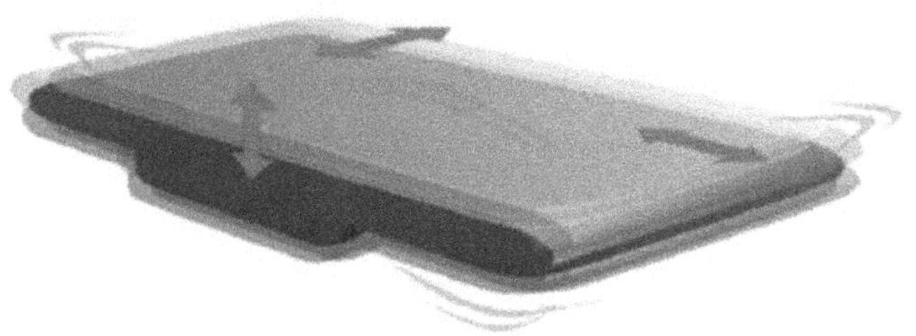

Table 2.1 *Technical Requirements for Vibration therapy platform*

Technical Requirements for VT Platform	
Frequency:	**20-50Hz**
Duration:	**0-120s**
Pause time:	**0-120s**
Intensity:	**low – high**
Repetition:	**1-20**

6

EFFECTS

Effects I

Table 2.2 *Effects of vibration therapy on Muscles*

Muscles
Vibration plate triggers reflexes
Subconscious → Reflexes cannot be controlled
Increased recruitment of muscle fibres:
Vibration Plate: 90-100%
Normal: 60-70%
High performance sports: 80-90%
Example: Muscle Atrophy
(MS, Confinement to bed,Incontinency)

Table 2.3 *Effects of vibration therapy on tendon/connective tissue*

Tendon/Connectivity Tissue
Tissues taking on vibrations alternatively
Friction of different tissues against each other releasing tissue adherences
Improved blood circulation

Effects II

Table 2.4 *Effects of vibration therapy on blood vessels*

Blood Vessels
1. Improved mobility of blood vessels
2. Improved circulation
3. Improved metabolic function → faster rregeneration
Example: Intermittent Claudication

Table 2.5 *Effects of vibration therapy on Hormones*

Hormones
1. VT influences the hormonal system positively
2. Increased distribution of growth-hormones
3. Increase of testosterone
4. Increased production of neurotrophin
5. Decreased production of cortisol

Effects III

Table 2.6 *Effects of vibration therapy on capsule and joints*

Capsule & Joints
1. Balance (Vestibular system)
2. **proprioception**, the process by which the body can vary muscle contraction in immediate response to incoming information regarding external forces
3. Improved neuro muscular connection
Example: High performance sports

Table 2.7 *Effects of vibration therapy on nerves and neurotransmitters*

Nerves/Neurotransmitters
1. Activation of Spinal reflexes
2. "Tuning" of the Nervous system via mobilisation/sensibilization
3. Increased number of Neurotransmitters (Dopamine/Serotonin) → Increase neuromuscular connections
Example: M. Parkinson

Effects IV

Table 2.8 *Effects of vibration therapy on bones and cartilage*

Bones & Cartilage
1. Bones follow the same rules as muscles
2. Speed of deformation strengthens the bones → Build-up of bones
Example: Osteoporosis
Intermittent pressure improves cartilage function···→ Increased synovial fluids surrounding cartilage (Improved nutrition)

Table 2.9 *Effects of vibration therapy on skin*

Skin
1. combination muscle, blood circulation, improved lymphatic transport, connective tissue causes a tightening of the skin

Table 2.10 *Vibration training as a complement*

Vibration training as a complement
1. VT causes mechanical vibrations which are transferred to the body
2. VT is a new and modern form of training because of its positive effects on different systems of the body
3. Used as warm-up, Strength training, Coordination training, Balance training, Regeneration, Cool-down
4. Excellent alternative to all sports

Table 2.11 *Vibration Training in therapy*

Vibration training in therapy
1. Absolute contra-indications: → Cardiac pace maker → Pregnancy → Cemented joint implants
2. Relative contra-indications: → Therapist needs to decide whether VT is indicated or not

Table 2.12 *Vibration training in sports*

Vibration training in sports
1. Improved coordination (central/peripheral NS) → Improved learning situation
2. Increased recruitment of muscle fibres (Intramuscular coordination) → Increased strength

3. Frequency of training: 3/week Eventually combined with strength training (super compensation) 4. Warm-up prior to endurance training → immediate ideal effects (increased efficiency)

Table 2.13 *Application areas of vibration training*

Application area
Medical Area 1. physical therapists, rehab clinics
Professional Area 2. sports consultants, sports clubs, training centers, golf clubs, tennis clubs
Fitness Area 3. fitness studios, wellness hotels

Table 2.14 *Application Fields of vibration training*

Application fields
Medical application Incontinence, osteoporosis, MS, rehabilitation following injuries, treatment of pain and stiffness
Professional application Effective exercising method for both hobby and serious athletes, stretches, extends and smooth muscles, increasing explosive strength, strength training.
Fitness application Improving coordination and movement ability eases tension

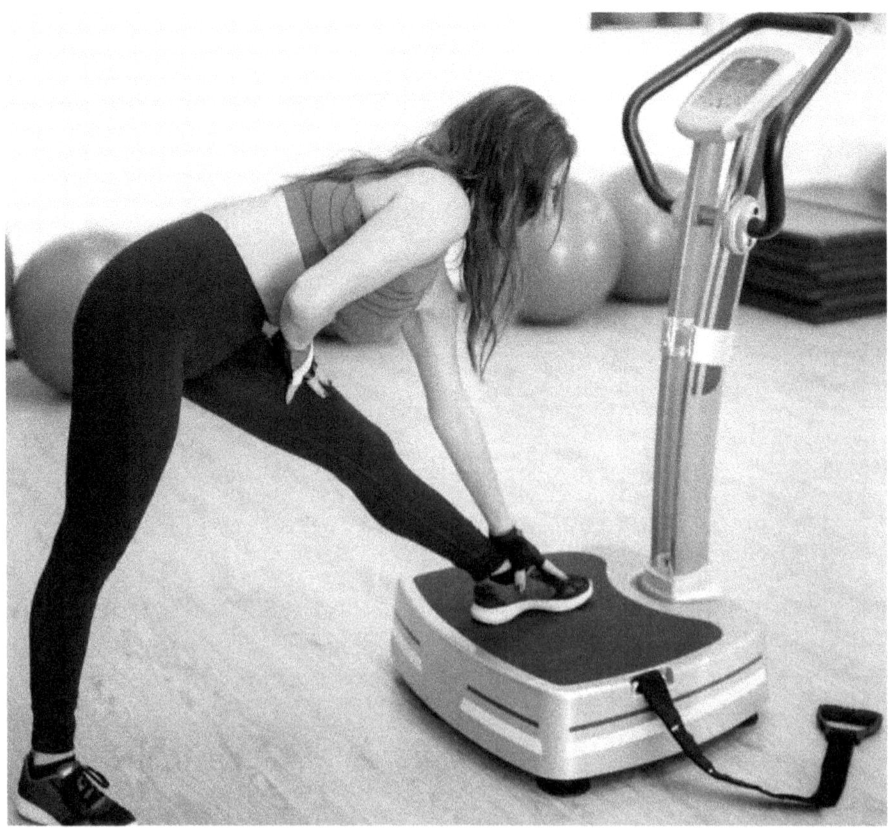

Fig 2.8 Stretching of Hamstring muscle on vibration platform

7

WHOLE BODY VIBRATION THERAPY IN OSTEOPOROSIS

Whole Body Vibration therapy is a promising treatment for people with Osteoporosis. Finding ways to reverse stop, or slow deterioration of the bones or even increase bone mass is critical to combating osteoporosis. Low-impact whole body vibration delivers mechanical loading to the skeleton, which can increase bone mass and improve balance.

One study tested 70 people post menopause with two 10-minute sessions of Whole body vibration therapy each day for 1 year. Most participants lost bone mass in that time, but those weighing less than 143 pounds increased bone mass density by 3.3%.

Another study in people after menopause tested 86 individuals for 6 months, utilizing 10-minute sessions five times per week. Bone mass density increased by 4.3% after treatment compared to a control group.

An analysis of 25 studies concluded that there were small but significant improvements in balance and gait speed among older adults after Whole body vibration therapy.

Research is ongoing, but studies have shown **mixed results on the use of vibration therapy for osteoporosis. Whereas some research shows significant change for bone mineral density in mature persons, other research shows no change at all.**

Fall prevention is especially important for those with osteoporosis. According to the Centers for Disease Control and Prevention (CDC) Trusted Source, falls are the leading cause of death for those over age 65.

As mentioned previously, positive outcomes of vibration therapy have been noted for improving balance and preventing falls in older adults.

Researchers debate factors such as how progressed a diagnosis of osteoporosis is, the level of intensity, whether WBV or LIV is more suitable, and how long treatments should last.

The most promising and consistent results Trusted **about vibration therapy for** osteoporosis stem from LIV.

Still, most research trusted source **concludes that vibration therapy will slow the progression of osteoporosis-related bone deterioration, even if it doesn't improve bone mineral density.**

Weight bearing exercise, adequate vitamin D, and a well-balanced diet are some factors that help maintain bone health. Vibration therapy has many benefits and may also help prevent the deterioration of bone, which is useful in the prevention of osteoporosis.

Vibration therapy may be a viable adjunct treatment option for those living with osteoporosis, especially in when it comes to maintaining balance, increasing muscle mass, and preventing falls. Still, the research is inconclusive regarding whether vibration therapy can increase bone density over time.

Various Positions on the vibration platform for Geriatric population and youngsters

8

VIBRATION THERAPY FOR THE YOUNG AND OLD

Not just for athletes or those concerned about fitness, vibration therapy exercises have powerful effects on muscle power.

As we age, our muscle power reduces making us less stable on our feet therefore increasing the risk of falls. With its very low stress on the cardiovascular system, vibration therapy is a great way for elderly patients to improve their balance and mobility.

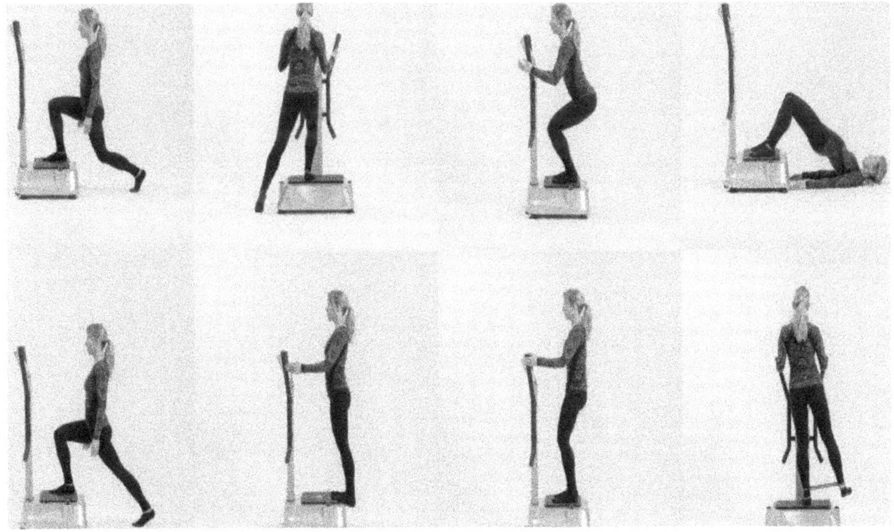

Fig 2.9 *Various Exercise Positions on the vibration platform*

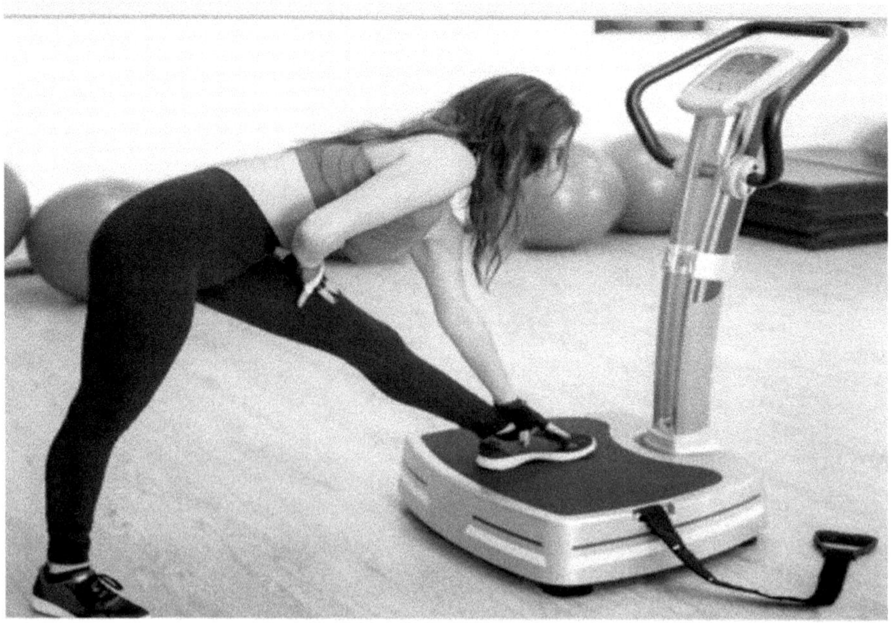

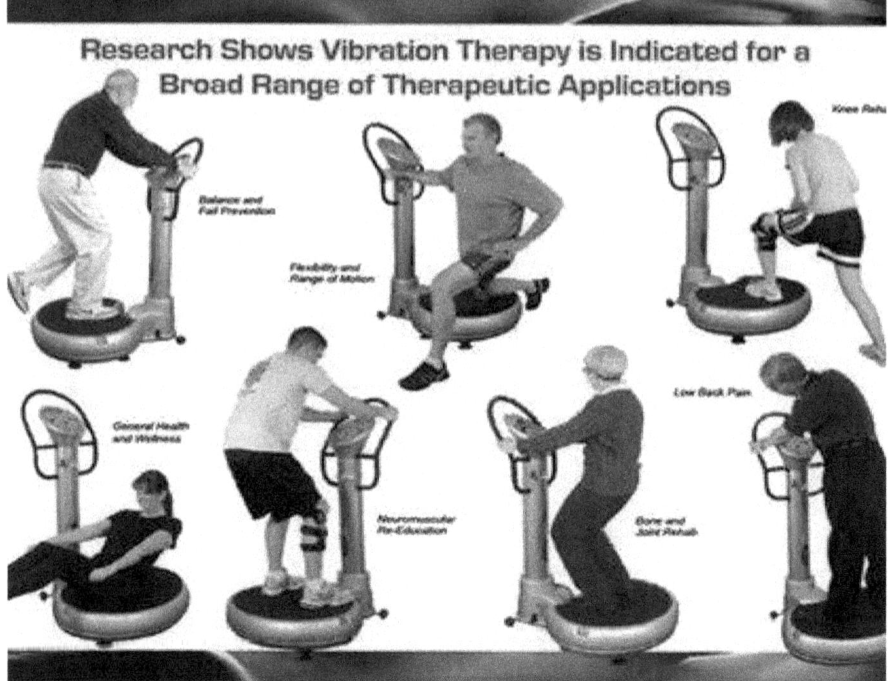

Fig 2.10 *Various Positions on the vibration platform for Geriatric population*

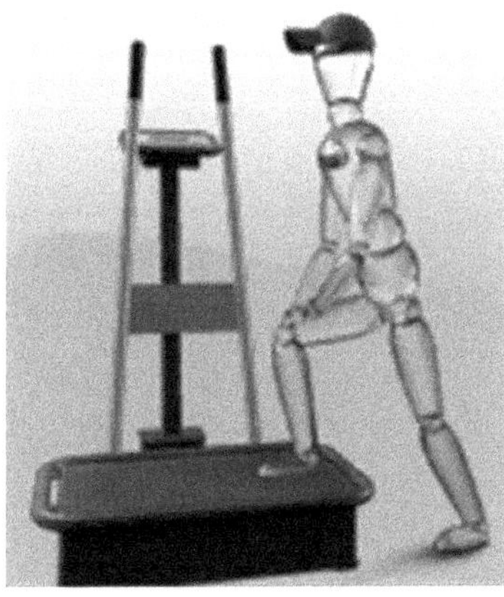

Bend one leg,

Standing on the plate.

Push hips forward.

Change legs

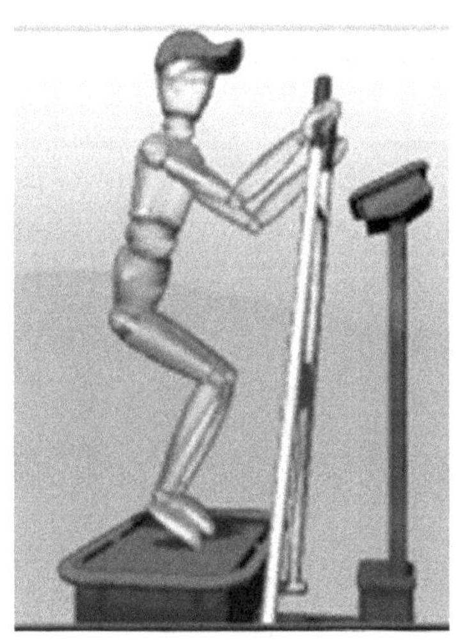

Feet hip wide,

Standing on the toes.

Knees slightly bent, not in

Front of the toes.

Pull abdomen up

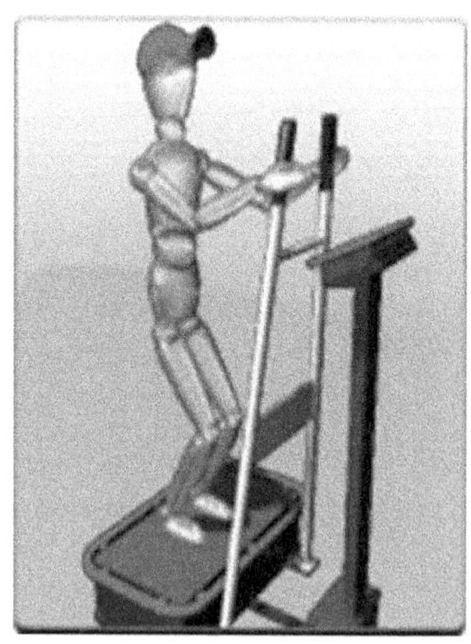

Stand with slightly bended knees

on the vibration platform

Push hips forward.

Create tension and release.

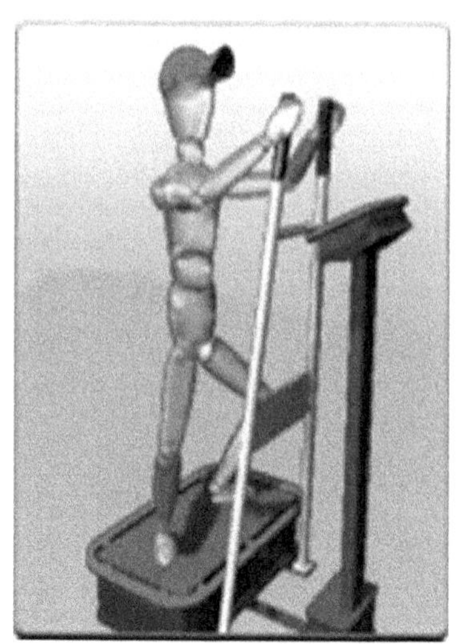

Stand wide on the plate.

Lift the heels altering.

Upper body is static

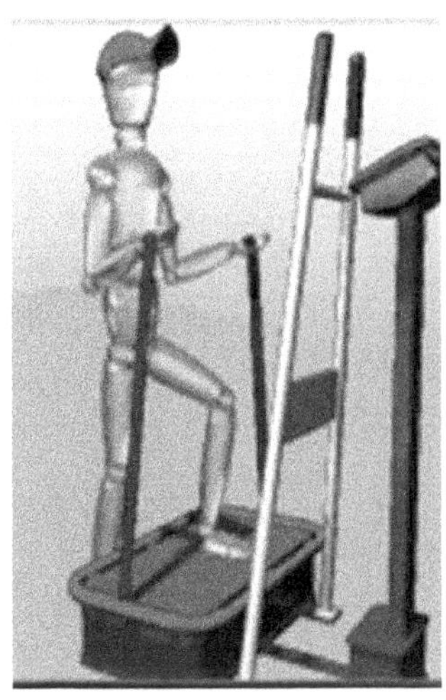

Put one leg on the vibration platform.

Pull the straps in a right angle. Palm is showing up.

Long straight spine. Abdomen is pulled in and up.

Change legs

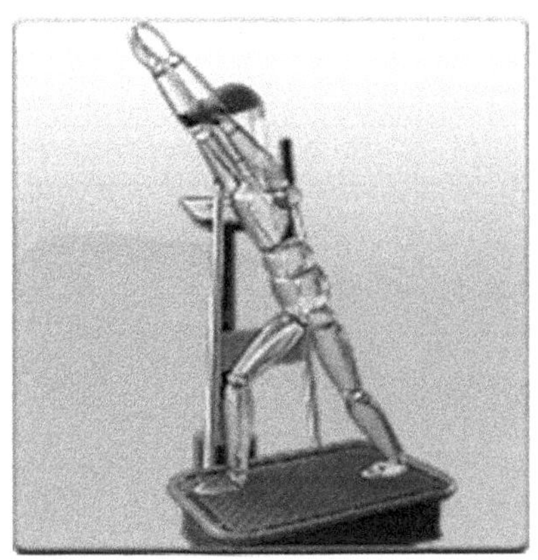

Stand in lunge on the vibration platform.

Upper body is lowered slightly

With straight spine. Straight arms,

Thumbs showing to the ceiling.

Change sides

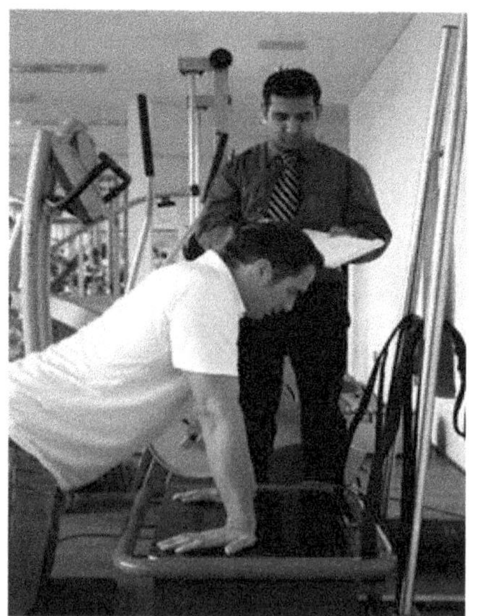

Golfers elbow

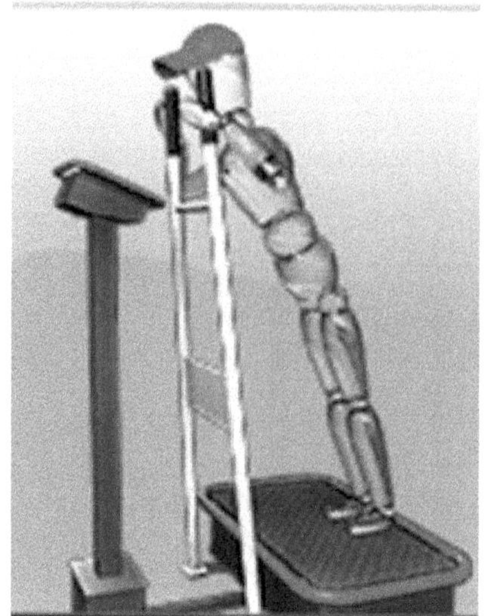

Calf stretch

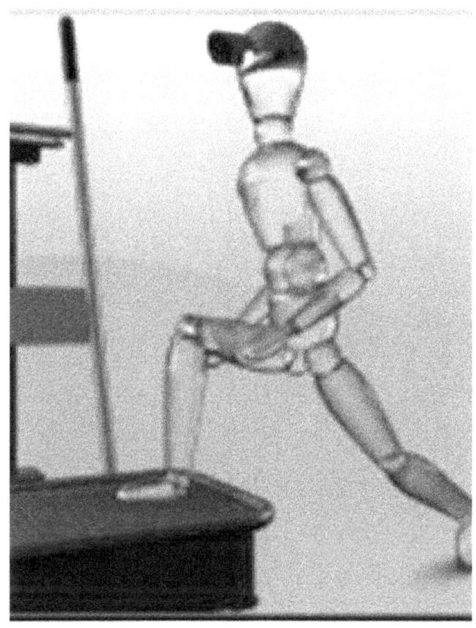

Single leg stance

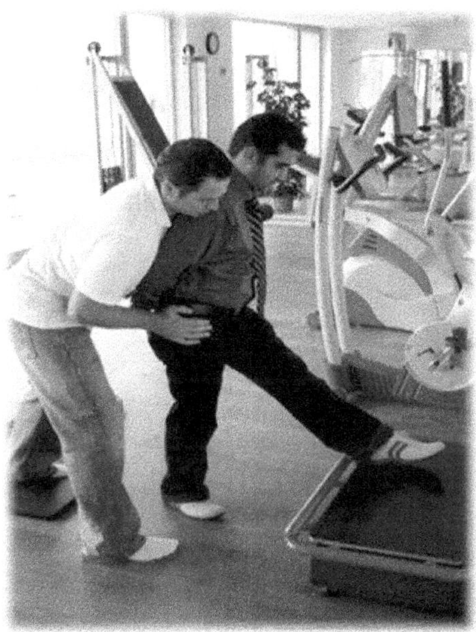

Hamstring stretch

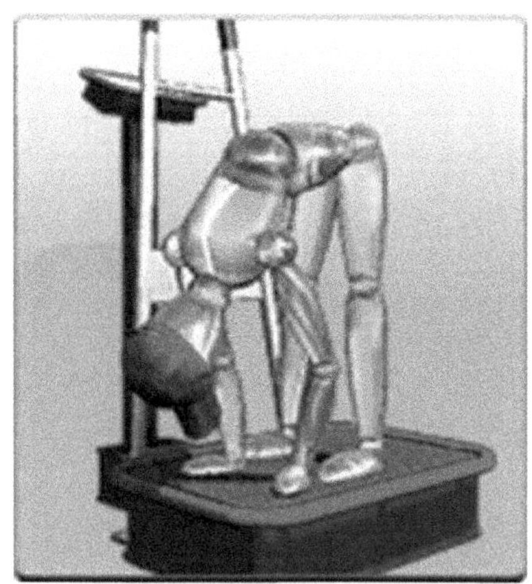

Spinal stretch

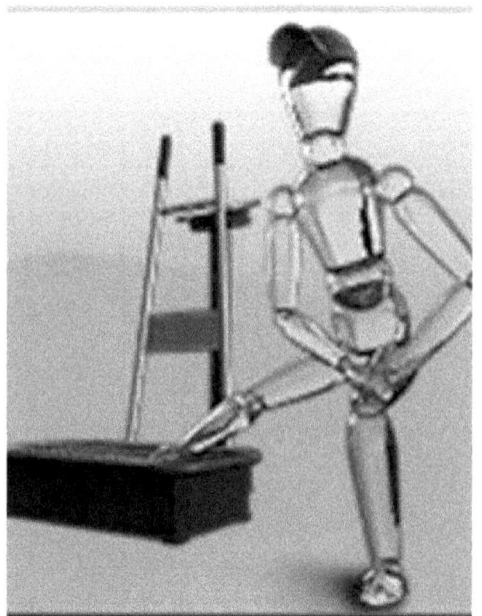

Adductor stretch

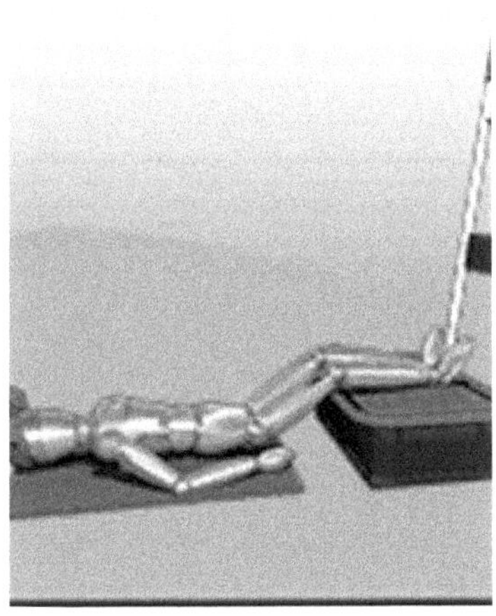

Calf relaxing

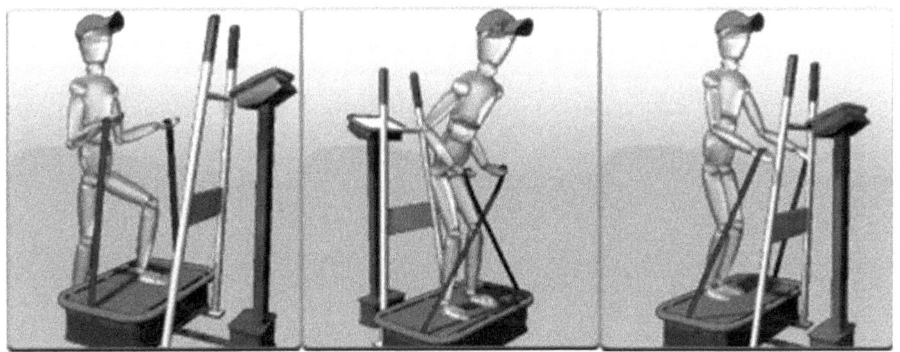

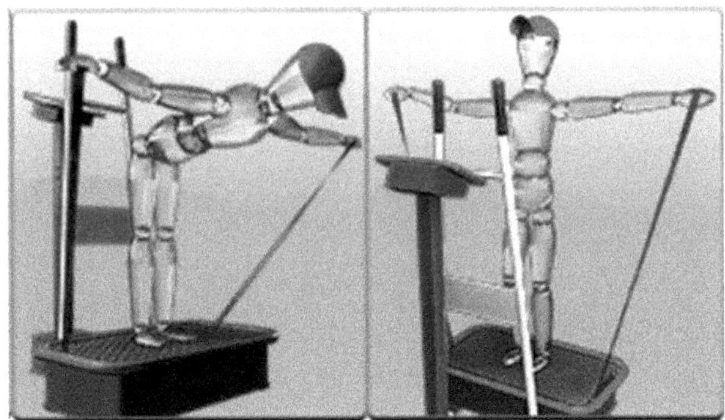

Using TheraBand

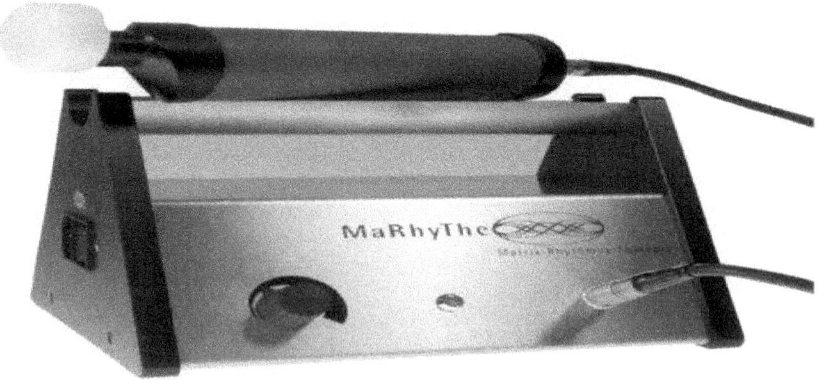

Fig 2.11 *Matrix Rhythm Therapy device*

9

THE MATRIX RHYTHM THERAPY CONCEPT

In the period 1989-1997 the research project "Clinically Linked Basic Research" was carried out at Erlangen University with support from the foundation "Stifterverband fur die Deutsche Wissenschaft" and the Ruth and Klaus Bahlsen Foundation. The therapeutic conclusion from the research was that cell processes must activate as much as possible on a systemic level in order to achieve healing. That means by changing the cellular environment.

Turning these insights into practice led to the Matrix Concept. In 1996 the concept of "Matrix Rhythm Therapy" was introduced and gained scientific recognition. This concept expressed the fact that every intervention on a cell – whether preventative, curative, regenerative or also destructive – works primarily via cell's environment, that is via the extracellular matrix. That is where the therapeutic action has its primary effect, which then leads in turn to effects on the cell.

Examined more closely, living structures consist of processes which constantly form and transform themselves: within a time span of about seven years the body replaces the entirety of its molecular constituents.

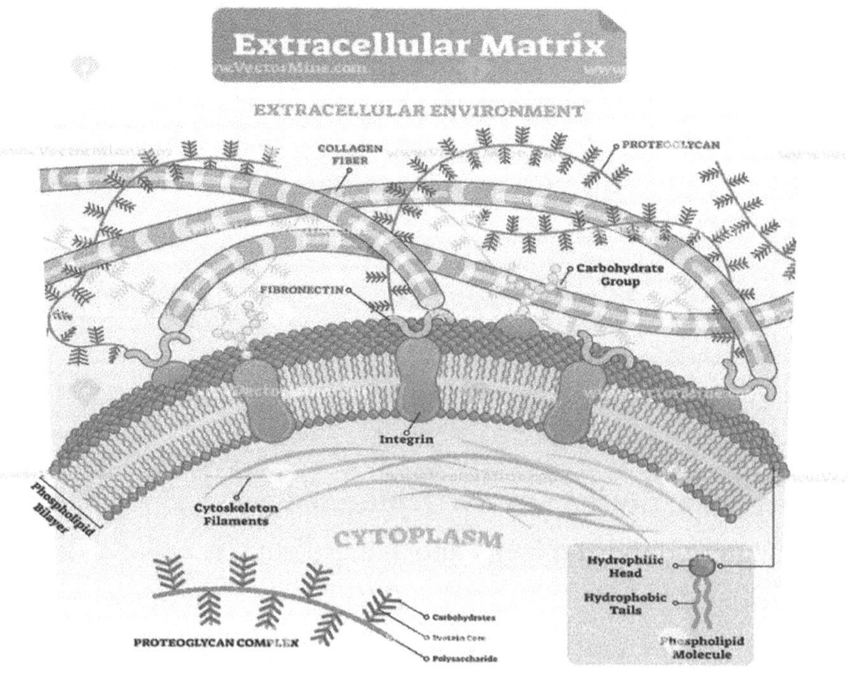

Fig 2.12 *Extra cellular Matrix*

The concept of Matrix Rhythm Therapy is based on the following essential points:

1. The skeletal musculature is our organ of locomotion.
2. As the biggest "clock-pulse generator" in the organism it plays the essential role, together with the heart, in the transport of fluids and the microcirculation in the organism.
3. The skeletal musculature has a specific rhythm. Its frequency spectrum, which is manifested in synchronous vibrations ranging from the physiological tremor to trembling and shivering, lies in the range of 8 to 12 Hz.

4. Pains are disturbances of cell processes. If cells do not have the proper surroundings and are not adequately supplied, then there are energy deficits and hardening occurs as a result.

5. When the mechanism of entrainment (entrainment signifies the synchronization of cells, organs and organisms by external rhythm) induces muscle cells to pulsate in the proper manner, this optimizers the cell logistics.

6. In addition, the supply of oxygen and heat, trace elements, vitamins, electrolytes and nutrients help to optimize the external environment of the cells.

7. Dr. Randoll recommends four basic modules for matrix Rhythm therapy: Rhythm, heat, oxygen and nutrition. It is important to inform the patient and involve the patient actively in the therapeutic process.

10

EXTRA CELLULAR MATRIX

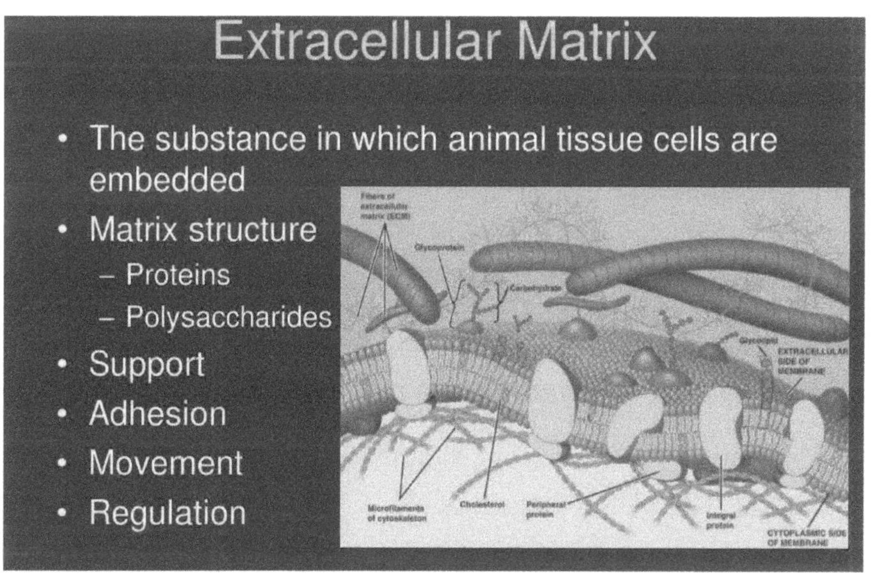

Fig 2.13 *Extra cellular matrix*

A FUNDAMENTAL PRINCIPLE: FIRST MICRO- EXTENSION THEN MACRO- MOBILIZATION

The treatment describes above generates microscopic stretching movements (rhythmic micro-extensions). The contraction residues are eliminated. The elasticity of the muscle is restored by activating the metabolism on the microscopic level. The cellular logistics are restored and we can move our muscles more freely again. A gradual transition to the next phase of the therapy follows: the macro mobilization of the muscle by the therapist.

Matrix rhythm therapy has proved to be effective in all cases where the symptoms are caused by disturbances in the microcirculation. Since its development at Erlangen University, this therapy approach has become standard in very many areas – especially in the perioperative domain, in trauma surgery, in rehabilitation, in pain therapy as well as the treatment of chronic diseases of the nervous system, skeletal and locomotor systems.

An additional field of application is prevention. Establishing optimal cell logistics effectively prevents illnesses and increases the body's resistance in injury.

ELIMINATE PAIN SYMPTOMS BY RELAXING THE MUSCLE?

Even among specialists today muscle contraction is still seen as the main energy-consuming process. Is this true?

Examining the functioning of muscle cells, we discover: In order to contract, a muscle cell must first have built up an energy potential on its membrane. When the impulse arrives from the nerve this potential breaks down and results in the tensing or contraction of the muscle. Thus from the standpoint of the muscle cell: tensing is a passive act. In contrast, restoring the energy potential once more –repolarization- and thereby the relaxed state of the muscle, is an active process which requires energy.

Living processes are characterized by phases of tension and relaxation. Muscles can be consciously tensed and relaxed. But due to insufficient energy, residual contraction and tissue adhesions can remain even after voluntary relaxation. These residues can no longer be eliminated by conscious action. Even intensive and deep meditation or yoga doesn't help. The muscles become rigid. Intervention from the outside is necessary to bring about the completely relaxed state, by stimulating the metabolism and restoring cellular logistics. Therefore activating the process of relaxation by intervening from the outside became the key to an effective therapy.

THE SUCCESS FORMULA: HEALTHY RHYTHMS

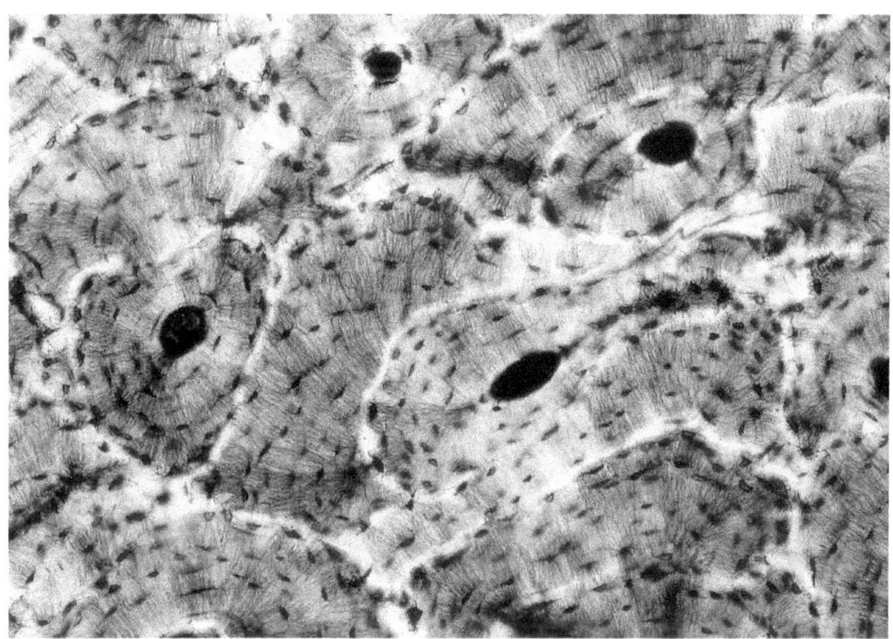

Fig 2.14 *Microscopic view of a tissue*

Rhythms are the key to a healthy life. The physiological role of the skeletal musculature and trembling of the muscles is generally accepted. Hence in the context of our systematic investigation of body rhythms we concentrated on the skeletal musculature. Do all people tremble in the same way?

In all people healthy muscles vibrate in the frequency range of 8 to 12 Hz. This can be observed directly on the cellular level. Muscle cells pulsate. What happens when the rhythm of pulsation changes? It can be shown with the help of piezoelectric sensors that muscle pulsation frequencies which lie outside the 8-12Hz range correlate positively with pains, muscle tension and other health problems. Changed muscle elasticity and plasticity are linked to changes in pulsation frequency and in the logistics of the living process on the cellular level.

11

RHYTHMS SHAPE PROCESSES

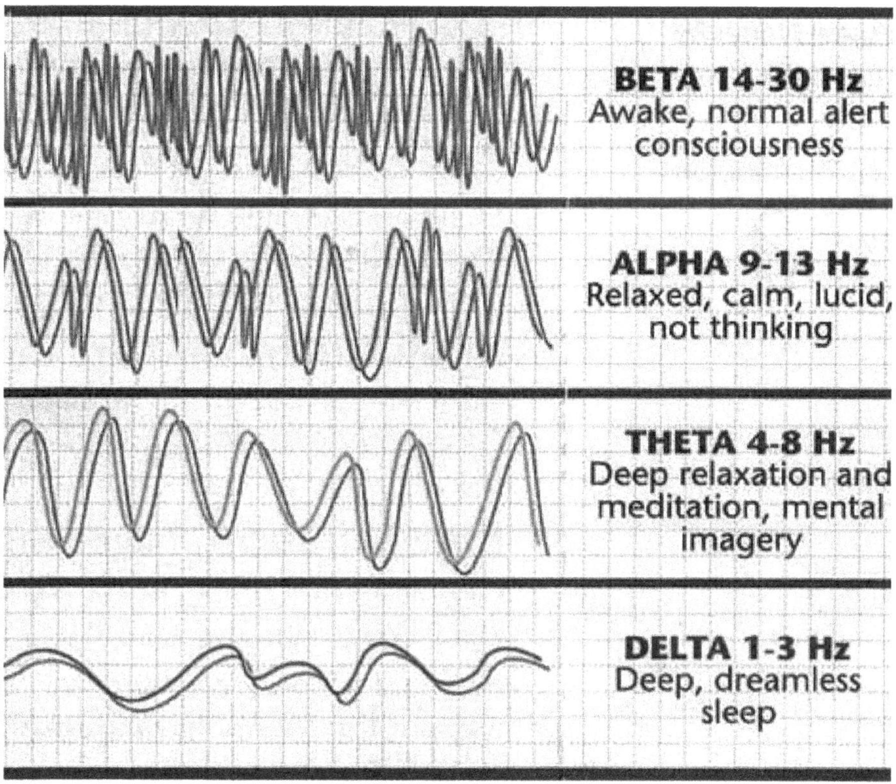

Fig 2.15 *Different Rhythms within the human body*

In fact, rhythmical processes are found in every living organism which has been studied up to now, including even single-celled organisms. Rhythms are essential structure-generating information, which can be destabilized or stabilized by outside influences.

In humans we can immediate recognize a variety of life processes that are rhythmic in character. The most obvious are breathing and heartbeat.

The octave principle in body rhythms:

Table 2.15 *Physiological Rhythms in Human Body*

Frequency of the heart	50 to 100 pulses per minute
Frequency of breathing	12 to 20 breaths per minute
Brain frequencies	
Beta	13 to 30 Hz
Alpha	8 to 12 Hz
Theta	4 to 7 Hz
Delta	0.5 to 3 Hz
Frequency of skeletal musculature	8 to 12 Hz

In biological systems there are never rigidly fixed frequencies, but only frequency ranges. This variability permits adaption and is essential to the survival of the organism.

Human beings are not independent from rhythms but must live in harmony with them. This understanding of the role of rhythms can be utilized therapeutically.

LIKE FISH IN WATER: CELLS IN THE EXTRACELLULAR MATRIX

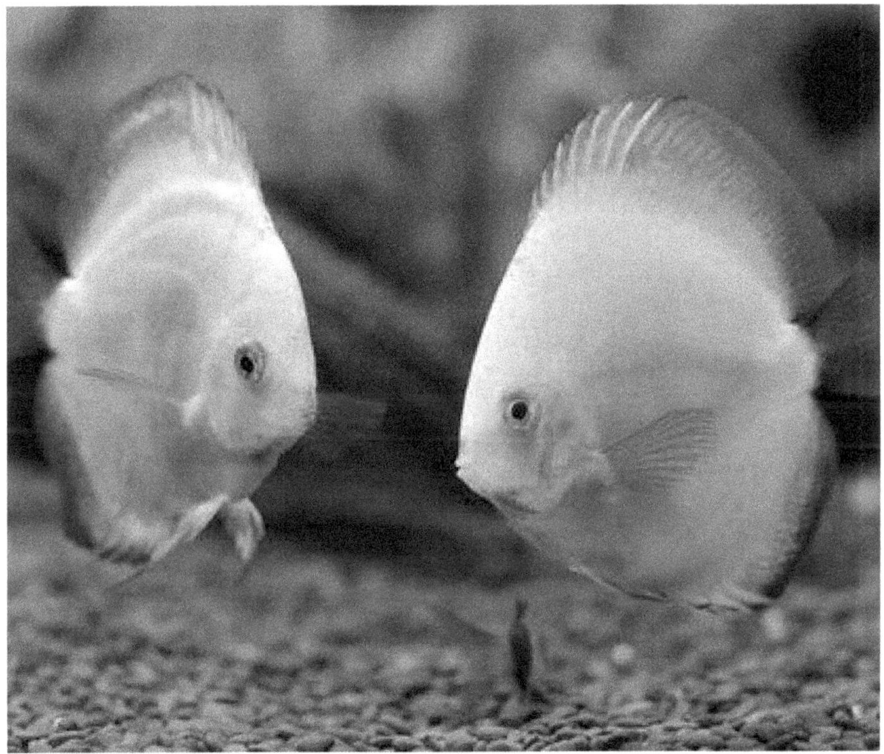

Fig 2.16 Fishes In the fresh water

The human body is a complex system. It consists of 70 trillion cells. These cells are all surrounded by the extra cellular matrix. All exchange and communication, all transport to and from the cells takes place through this matrix. There is no other possibility to reach the cell other than via this transit pathway. The extracellular matrix pervades the entire organism.

Cells are dependent on the special environment in which they have developed and to which they have adapted themselves. Hence the state and the quality of this extracellular medium is a determining factor for our health.

Sticking with the metaphor of the fish, we can say: like fish in water, the cells in our body are surrounded by the extracellular matrix. The vital logistics of supply and removal of all substances occurs via that medium.

The wellbeing of each cell thus depends on its surroundings, just as the wellbeing of fish depends on the quality of the water they are swimming in.

These considerations suggest a therapeutic approach focused on the "habitat" of the cell.

Entrainment means gently inviting the tissue to "swing along"

Entrainment signifies the synchronization of cells, organs and organism by an external rhythm. Matrix rhythm therapy applies the normal physiological muscle frequency from the outside, in order to readapt derailed cellular and extracellular processes. In the fields of osteopathy, manual medicine and other physiotherapeutic techniques this effect of MaRhyThe has been recognized and has become an integral part of therapeutic practice in many places.

Matrix rhythm therapy enables the therapist to treat even the deeper layers of tissue in a directed, specific and gentle way. The goal is a pain-free mode of treatment. Pain evokes corresponding defense reactions and leads to further tension and cramping. This is why a gentle treatment is especially important.

Sustained therapeutic success comes when tissue elasticity and plasticity has been achieved in the relaxed state. This "reset" correlates positively with a favorable supply status of the cells and is the ideal preparation for renewed training programs.

WHY IS MATRIX RHYTHM THERAPY SO EFFECTIVE?

Experts have pointed out that system- optimizing is the goal. But not simply in terms of optimizing individual system parameters. "Resource Management" is required. This occurs indirectly, i.e. inductively. Therapists are process- optimizers for suitable, often personalized contexts.

According to the Matrix Concept, therapists utilize the Matrixmobil both locally and systemically. They aim to stimulate healing processes via entrainment by acting directly on the cell biological level.

Matrix therapists pass on their knowledge and experience to their mature patients. These patients know that Matrix Rhythm Therapy can only stimulate the natural healing powers of their own bodies. The patient recognizes his or her active task, which often means giving up cherished habits of living. The patient is solely responsible for maintaining his or her newly- recovered health by organizing daily life accordingly.

What the therapist does is above all to create favorable conditions on the cellular level. The patient is responsible for maintenance of health and prevention via changed behavior in the areas of nutrition, exercise and relaxation.

Working with the physiological frequency and amplitude range is a unique feature of Matrix Rhythm Therapy

From the historical standpoint Matrix Rhythm Therapy is a vibrational treatment focused on the skeletal musculature. In the broadest sense it can be seen as future development of classical vibration massage. Vibration massages are effective methods in the area of rehabilitation and sports. They are naturally very strenuous for the therapist and are limited by their relative inability to access deeper lying tissue.

The reason for the success of Matrix Rhythm Therapy lies in its approach based on cell biology. Matrix Rhythm Therapy stimulates the natural rhythm and indirectly regulates the processes which are coupled to that rhythm. While many treatment methods work with rigidly fixed frequencies, Matrix Rhythm Therapy utilizes the whole "window" of physiological frequencies, thereby allowing the flexible tissue to adapt in a healthy way.

12

THE MATRIXMOBIL – THE EXTENDED ARM OF THE THERAPIST

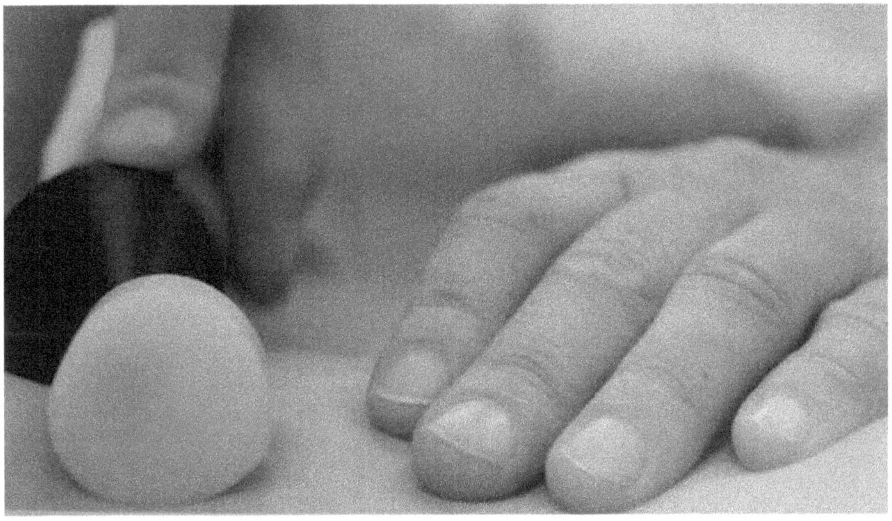

Fig 2.17 *Matrix Rhythm Therapy Device in action*

Matrix Rhythm Therapy was developed as a logical consequence of the observation of physiological rhythms, and of measurements carried out on the musculature of the subjects with various different symptomatic conditions. The result was a therapy method which works in conformity with nature. Subsequently the Matrixmobil was created as a therapeutic device. The working head of this device, the resonator, functions essentially as the extended arm of the therapist. First the tissue elasticity is explored via the resonator. Hardenings of the muscle tissue are detected and localized. In the second step the therapist applies haptic skills and detailed anatomical knowledge to treat process derailments in a precisely targeted way.

HOW DOES THIS WORK?

Firstly the Matrixmobil is applied to the surface of the patient's body. By means of the specially shaped resonator head the trained therapist propagates phase – synchronized magneto – mechanical vibrations deep into the body tissue. In this way the musculature in various layers is acted upon in the physiological frequency range. The applied vibration is modulated between 8 and 12 Hz. Among other things, this generates asymmetric pressure in the tissue, which stimulates the pumping and sucking effects of the tissue's own vibrations. The nerve endings are stimulated and the whole tissue is readjusted to its proper rhythm.

13

Z-VIBES

AN APPROACH TOWARDS ORAL SENSORY MOTOR REHABILITATION

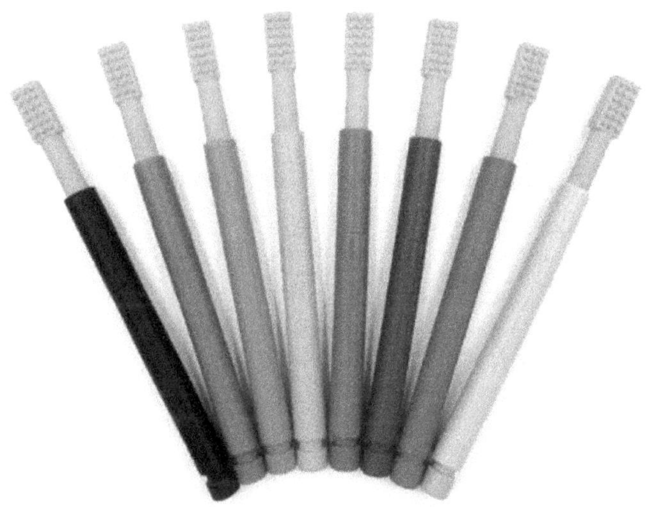

The Z-Vibe is a vibratory oral motor tool that can help build oral tone and improve a variety of speech, feeding, and sensory skills. Use it to provide a varied sensory experience and/or to provide targeted tactile cues within the oral cavity. Its gentle vibration provides a new level of sensory stimulation to increase oral focus and draw more attention to the lips, tongue, cheeks, and jaw. Vibration can also be very calming, soothing, and organizing. The Z-Vibe's sleek, innovative design features a lightweight, textured plastic handpiece. The texture around the handle provides a slip-proof grip, and it can also be brushed along the cheeks, arms, hands, etc. for additional tactile input. The handle comes with a blue Probe Tip on one end and a Switch Tip on the other. Use the Probe Tip for oral motor assessment and development. This end of the handle is sealed off from the internal components so that no saliva, water, or moisture can compromise the unit from that end. To turn the unit on, simply twist the Switch Tip at the opposite end of the handle just until the unit starts to vibrate (please do not over-tighten!). This end of the handle is open so that you can easily replace the battery when necessary.

PHARYNGEAL-ORAL FUNCTION AND SPEECH PRODUCTION

The oral-pharyngeal region serves multiple functions: sucking, swallowing, respiration, speech, and mastication, as well as gagging, vomiting, coughing, and snoring. These functions involve the large jaw muscles, the smaller jaw-opening muscles, and muscles of the face, lips, cheeks, tongue, palate, and pharynx.

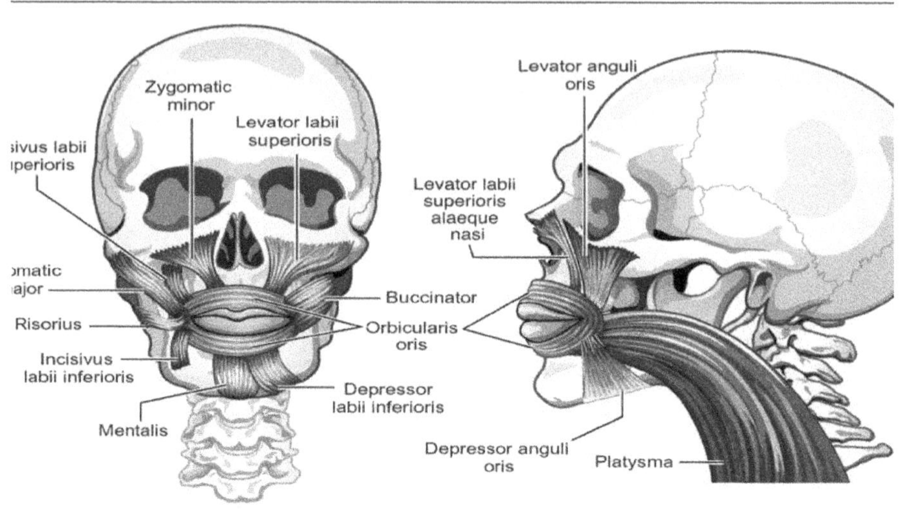

Why is oral motor therapy important

To achieve a right pose in yoga several muscle groups work together in a delicate balance of strength, coordination , movement, and endurance.

Speech & feeding are very much same, only localized to the muscles of the lips, tongue, jaws, and cheeks.

In order to properly articulate sounds and manage food, the mouth muscles need to be in very specific "poses"

Where does the Z-Vibe come in

The Z-Vibe is a tool to help you provide targeted tactile cues within the oral cavity without getting your fingers in harm's way.

It also takes tactile learning to the next level with the added bonus of vibration.

The gentle vibration of the Z-Vibes provides added sensory stimulation to increase oral focus and draw more attention to the articulators.

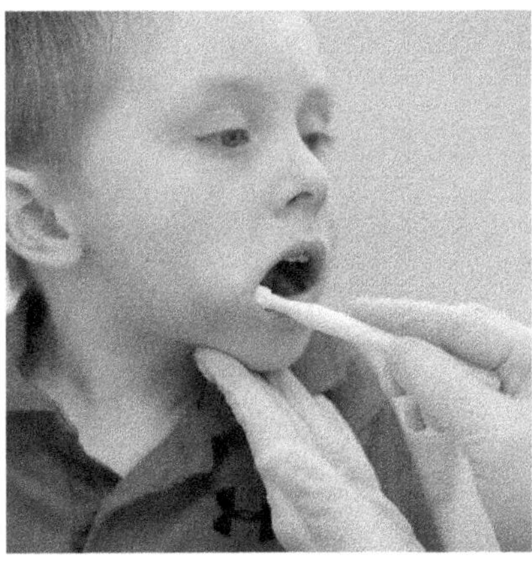

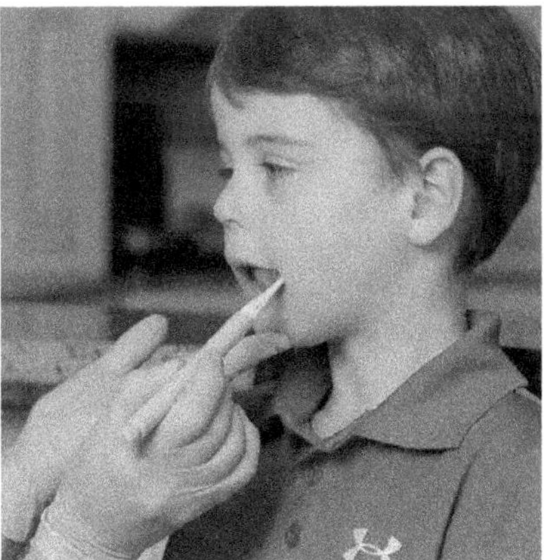

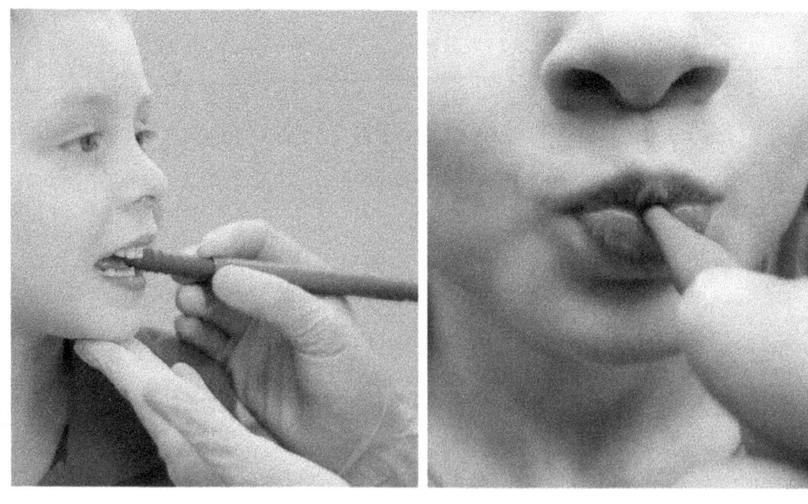

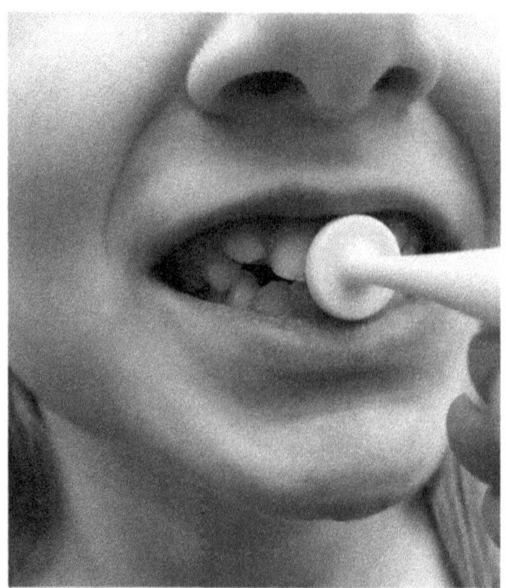

ORAL MOTOR EXERCISES WITH THE Z-VIBE

Posted by Debra C. Lowsky, MS, CCC-SLP on 20th May 2013

What is oral motor therapy?

Oral motor therapy works on the oral skills necessary for proper speech and feeding development. For example, try saying "la la la" right now, paying attention to what your tongue is doing. In order to produce the /l/ sound, the tongue tip must elevate to the alveolar ridge (just behind the upper front teeth). It must also be able to function independently - or dissociate - from the jaw. Oral motor therapy works on these "pre-requisites" for speech and feeding.

WHY IS ORAL MOTOR THERAPY IMPORTANT?

Think about yoga. In order to get a pose right, several muscle groups must be working together in a delicate balance of strength, coordination, movement, and endurance. Speech and feeding are very much the same, only localized to the muscles of the lips, tongue, jaw, and cheeks. In order to properly articulate sounds and manage food, the mouth muscles need to be in very specific "poses." For example, try drinking from a straw right now and pay attention to what your mouth is doing - your lips should be pursed and closed around the straw, the tongue tense and retracted, and the cheeks taut. Most people naturally learn how to do this on their own. But some individuals (particularly those with developmental delays) need oral motor therapy to learn those skills.

WHERE DOES THE Z-VIBE COME IN?

Most people are either visual or auditory learners. Sometimes, however, these two senses are not enough, and we must look to the sense of touch. Imagine you're in a yoga class again. You've heard the instructor explain a pose, you've seen her demonstrate it, but it's just not clicking for you. So the instructor comes over and adjusts your arm into in the right position. Similarly, sometimes you need to physically show an individual where the tongue should go for this sound, that skill, etc. This is called giving them a tactile cue. The Z-Vibe is a tool to help you provide targeted tactile cues within the oral cavity without getting your fingers in harm's way.

It also takes tactile learning to the next level with the added bonus of vibration. The gentle vibration of the Z-Vibe provides added sensory stimulation to increase oral focus and draw more attention to the articulators.

BEFORE YOU START

Keep in mind that you may have to start slowly, gradually introducing the Z-Vibe. You absolutely do not have to use vibration, but it is there if the individual needs more input. For more tips on using vibration with the Z-Vibe, click here.

For individuals with hypo or hypersensitivities, you may have to work on normalizing oral sensation before proceeding with the following exercises.

The Z-Vibe comes with one Probe Tip. There are over 25 additional tip attachments available. Most of the exercises below can be done with the Probe Tip alone, but I mention some other possibilities as well.

LIP CLOSURE

Lip closure (also known as "lip seal") is the ability to close the lips around a spoon, cup, straw, lollipop, etc. It also prevents drooling and is required to pronounce the /p/b/m/ sounds.

- Place the handle of the Z-Vibe just under the nose. Gently press downward until the upper lip makes contact with the lower lip. Then place the handle just above the chin. Gently press upward until the lower lip makes contact with the upper lip. This helps establish the concept of lip closure.

- Place the Preefer Tip horizontally between the center of the lips. Instruct the individual to close his/her lips firmly around the tip and hold for 3-5 seconds. Make sure that the individual is not biting down on the tip. Follow up with the production of /p/b/m/ sounds. This exercise can also be done with the Probe Tip, Mini Tip, or Bite-n-Chew Tip (shown below with the Bite-n-Chew Tip XL).

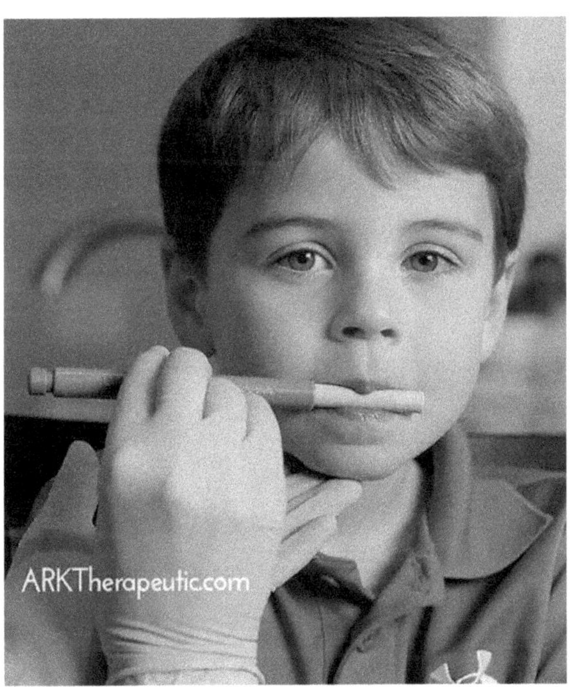

JAW GRADING

Try saying a long 'e' sound and compare that with the 'aw' sound. Or, imagine biting into a big sandwich versus a potato chip. Can you feel the height difference? This height difference is called jaw grading. It's the ability to visually judge how far the jaw should open for certain foods and vowel sounds.

- Use the bite blocks on the backs of the Animal Tips to practice jaw grading. The Dog Tip has the thickest block; the Mouse Tip has a thinner one; and the Cat Tip has the thinnest. Beginning with the Dog Tip (which will be the easiest one), have the individual bite and hold the block for 3-4 seconds. Release and repeat. Progress to the Mouse Tip and then the Cat Tip. Skip to 1:25 of the video below to watch.
- Other parts of the Animal Tips can be used as well. The ears, cheeks, and faces all have varied shapes that will require the jaw to open to different heights.

TONGUE AND JAW DISSOCIATION

As mentioned before, the tongue and jaw must be able to move independently of one another for certain speech sounds. It's also required in order to lateralize the tongue and move food around inside the mouth.

- Place a Probe Tip or Bite-n-Chew Tip in between the pre-molars. Instruct the individual to bite down and hold. Then have him/her say "lalalalalalala." Relax and repeat. Biting down on the tip forces the tongue to move on its own without moving the jaw up and down.
- Instruct the individual to bite down on the tip again. This time, have him/her place the tongue tip on the alveolar ridge behind the upper front teeth. Then place it behind the bottom front teeth. Repeat several times.

- While biting down on the tip, instruct the individual to do a tongue pop. Suck the tongue up onto the roof of the palate and then pop it. Work up to 25 in a row.

TONGUE ELEVATION

Swallow right now, paying attention to your tongue as it lifts to make contact with the roof of the mouth. Now say "la la la," paying attention to your tongue tip elevating. Now do the same for "ga ga ga." The ability to elevate the tongue is an important skill for swallowing, manipulating food in the mouth, and producing certain speech sounds.

- Place the Tongue Tip vertically just in front of the mouth. Instruct the individual to place the tongue tip inside the hole. Gently guide the tongue up and down to establish the concept of tongue elevation. You can also guide the tongue from side to side for lateralization.
- Gently press the Probe/Mini Tip onto the back of the tongue and then up to the palate (this provides a tactile cue for the tongue to elevate). Remove the tip from the mouth and instruct the individual to produce the /k/g/y/ sounds.
- Hold the Z-Vibe vertically and apply gentle upward pressure to the alveolar ridge using the Fine Tip. Then remove the tip and instruct the individual to touch the same spot with his/her tongue tip. Follow up with the functional goal of tongue tip sounds /t/d/n/l/s/z/. This exercise can also be performed with the Probe/Mini Tips.

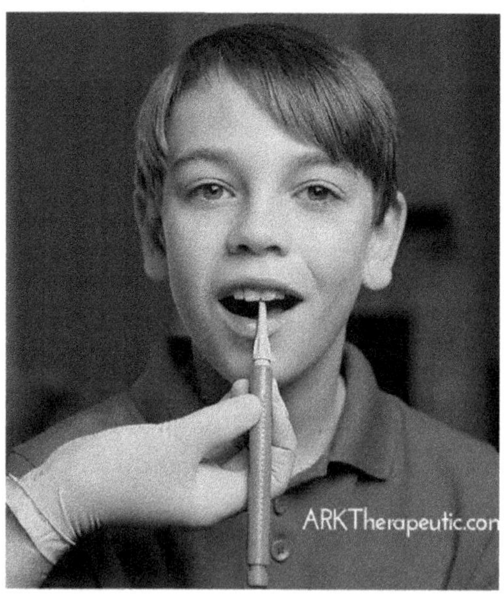

TONGUE LATERALIZATION

Tongue lateralization is the ability to move one's tongue from side to side, which is necessary for food manipulation, bolus formation, and the retrieval of leftover food particles from the mouth.

- Stroke one side of the tongue in a back-to-front movement using the Probe, Mini, or Fine Tip. Repeat on the other side.
- Gently push the tongue to the opposite side of the mouth with the Probe/Mini Tip. Repeat on the other side. This establishes the concept of moving the tongue from side to side. To increase the difficulty, instruct the individual to push against the tip for resistance.
- Place the Probe/Mini Tip inside the cheek area to one side. Have the individual touch it with the tip of his tongue. Repeat to the other side. Go back and forth several times to simulate lateralization.

14

VIBRATION GUN

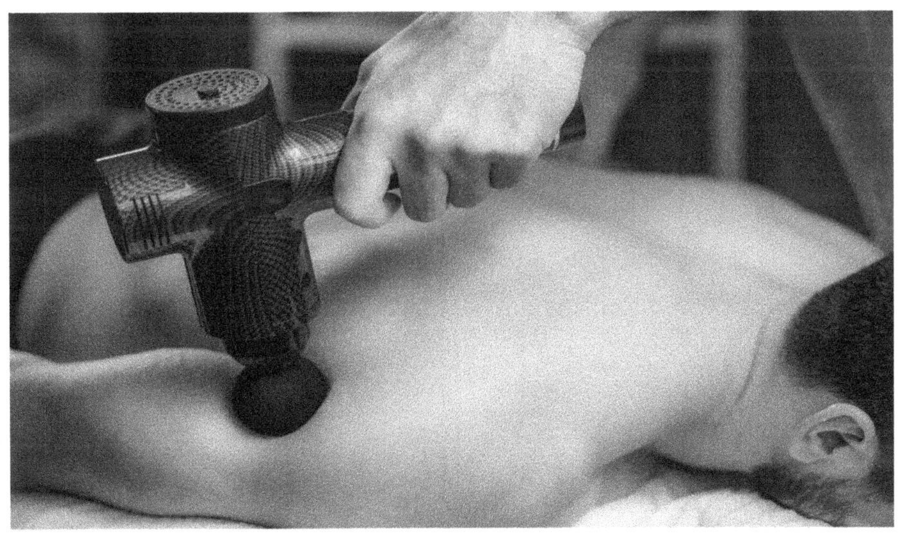

Massage guns can greatly improve muscle endurance, increase power, and improve kinesthetic awareness. The effects include decreased pain, improved muscle tone, range of motion, and circulation.

BENEFITS OF MASSAGE GUNS: PROS AND CONS

Massage guns have become widely popular and easy to obtain. Many swear by these small handheld devices, which operate differently than the old vibrating massage guns. The new wave of massage guns, such as the Theragun percussion gun, pulse in and out, percussing the tissue (and stimulating deeper). These recovery tools are used by physical therapists, athletes and individuals who work out to relieve pain and improve circulation.

BENEFITS OF PERCUSSION MASSAGE GUNS

Some of the physical benefits of massage and using a percussion massage gun include:

1. Reduced muscle tension
2. Improved circulation
3. Stimulation of the lymphatic system
4. Decreases soreness after workouts
5. Improved sports performance and muscle mass
6. Improved rehabilitation from injuries
7. Provides pain relief
8. Stimulates the nervous system
9. Facilitates lactic acid release
10. Increased mobility, flexibility, and pliability
11. Injury prevention
12. Breaks up scar tissue (potentially)

REDUCED MUSCLE TENSION

Primarily, the nerve pathways travel from our brain into our spinal cords, exiting the spinal cord through nerve roots and ultimately reaching a "target organ." A target organ can be muscles, blood vessels, digestive and hormone producing organs. This is called the efferent pathway with a primary function of directly facilitating or inhibiting skeletal muscles or smooth muscles in target organs. The sensory pathway travels from the target organs back through the nerve roots into the spinal cord and usually all the way up to the brain. This is called the afferent pathway.

Massage guns reduce muscle tension by bombarding the afferent or sensory pathway with a high intensity stimulus. The effect is similar to when one bumps one's elbow and instinctively rubs it.

There are many forms of therapeutic high intensity afferent stimulus. Moist heat, Ice, tape, massage, jacuzzi, foam rollers, joint manipulation and percussion massagers essentially work the same way. They bombard the nervous system with high intensity afferent (sensory) stimulus thus causing a reflexive inhibition of the muscle tension.

IMPROVED CIRCULATION

An equally important advantage of massage gun therapy is the improvement of circulation. Better blood circulation means better nutrients and oxygen supply within the body. The nutrients and oxygen are needed for tissue repair and efficient body function.

Massage guns, when used correctly, have demonstrated the ability to improve the blood flow within a section of your body. A full body massage with these devices may lead to better circulation throughout the body.

One mechanism is a reflexive relation of the smooth muscles in the arterial blood system as well as a relaxation of the muscles allowing for decreased resistance to circulation. Poor blood circulation has adverse effects on your overall health.

STIMULATION OF THE LYMPHATIC SYSTEM

Lymphatic stimulation may also improve from using a massage gun. The lymphatics is the third leg of your circulatory system. Arteries bring oxygen rich blood to the tissue, veins bring deoxygenated blood back to the heart and lungs to pick up oxygen, and the lymphatics circulate interstitial fluid back to the heart to be reabsorbed into the blood.

Massage gun therapy has the potential to stimulate lymph nodes which in turn may help circulate the lymphatic fluids to areas of the body where they are needed.

Your lymphatic system includes several lymph nodes that are placed throughout various areas of the human body. Lymph nodes are tucked away deep within the body or sometimes underneath the skin. The primary weapons these lymph nodes carry is known as lymphocyte. These nodes act as collection areas to store white blood cells (Lymphocytes) to fight potential infections within the body.

DECREASED SORENESS AFTER WORKOUTS

Anyone who works out or lifts weights knows that if you want to increase muscle strength and mass you must focus on increasing the stress systematically over time. The most common way to achieve this is to lift heavier weights or add volume over time. As we get more advanced, pushing the envelope means increased recovery needs over time. This sometimes can mean painful aches within the muscles known as Delayed Onset Muscle Soreness or DOMS. DOMS can last up to three days after a heavy workout.

Massage gun therapy can greatly reduce delayed onset muscle soreness (DOMS). This study from 2014 showed vibration therapy is an effective treatment for prevention and management of DOMS. Also, the evidence that vibration therapy improves muscular endurance and increases power may reduce DOMS overall by improving muscular adaptations over time.

Both compression and vibration therapies use the same mechanism for muscle recovery. However, percussive therapy works directly over muscle tissue and has the potential to provide much stronger, specific results. The current research on vibration therapy is a good indicator that percussive therapy may be a much more effective treatment option. If you are experiencing real-time muscle pain, percussive therapy can help by breaking up the pain signals sent by your brain to your body.

IMPROVED SPORTS PERFORMANCE AND MUSCLE MASS

Many professional athletes (Tom Brady being a prime example) endorse and use percussion guns for the benefits we have discussed earlier.

Both whole body and localized massage gun therapy have been shown to improve muscle mass and strength in older adults. Massage guns can greatly improve muscle endurance, increase power, and improve kinesthetic awareness.

The effects include decreased pain, improved muscle tone, range of motion, and circulation. Because massage guns are so effective, it is easier to recover more quickly, train more consistently and consequently perform better on the field, court, and pitch.

Efficient blood circulation and soft tissue mobility enhancements offered by percussive therapy may help the body perform at a higher level. Any athlete who is a top performer will tell you just how important it is to have a relaxed body before a big competition.

REHABILITATION – POST INJURY CARE

Percussion massagers are recommended for rehabilitation treatment. As physical rehabilitation specialists, we've seen this firsthand over many years:

Massage gun therapy is highly recommended for rehabilitation treatment because it not only hastens recovery but can also prevent re-injury. Massage gun use during rehabilitation is supplementary to the standard methods of rehabilitation therapy. This is achieved via improved healing and recuperation of atrophied or damaged muscles caused by trauma or illness.

Because percussion therapy facilitates efficient circulation within those areas (fascial tissues and muscles), flexibility is enhanced and the healing process is hastened.

The following are examples of conditions which are being treated more commonly using massage gun therapy

Muscle soreness

Sciatica

Muscle cramps and spasms

TMJ syndrome

Nonspecific low back pack

Shin Splints

Carpal Tunnel Syndrome

PAIN RELIEF

The percussion gun can also help in acute injuries where muscles are guarding an injured area as well as with chronic pain syndromes.

This technique is a natural way to decrease use of pain medication, injections, and other more invasive treatments. Always see a health care professional if you have any questions or concerns about an injury and the use of a percussion massage gun on an injured area.

NERVOUS SYSTEM STIMULATION

Nerve function is crucial if you want to lead a long and healthy life. Massage gun therapy can stimulate the nervous system and potentially improve certain essential functions.

One potential effect of percussive therapy is simulating production or release of the feel-good hormones such as serotonin and dopamine. Optimal levels of these chemicals mean sharper focus and a generally elevated mood.

FACILITATES LACTIC ACID RELEASE

Every athlete or gym enthusiast will tell you how frustrating it can be when you are working out and suddenly you feel tired, nauseated, and cramped. This intra- or post-workout unpleasantness occurs when there isn't enough oxygen in the body's muscles, which is essential to convert newly formed lactate into energy. As a result, lactic acid build-up happens faster than the body can burn it up.

A massage gun can help dispel the extra lactic acid into the circulatory system and get you going again. This also has the potential to reduce DOMS that may happen later.

IMPROVED MOBILITY OF MUSCLES/PLIABILITY OF TISSUE

Deep tissue massage provided by massage guns can help push out waste, improve blood circulation and release tension. This in turn helps improve tissue metabolism. This healthy exchange aids in preventing injuries and hastens tissue repair.

Improved tissue health will support more regular exercise, which will typically leads to improved flexibility. Massage guns are also frequently used while stretching to help improve the depth of stretch, potentially leading to improved muscle and joint flexibility.

INJURY PREVENTION

Massage guns can be used to prevent injury by increasing muscle temperature which increases pliability and flexibility. This accelerates warm-up and recovery, and contributes to reduced injury risk.

They can be used before a workout to wake up the muscles as a warm up. Massage gun therapy as a warm-up ensures that your muscles are supplied with enough oxygen and activation before starting exercise.

POTENTIALLY BREAKS UP SCAR TISSUE

There are accounts, though not backed up by scientific research, that massage gun therapy can be effective in reducing scar tissue. More importantly, percussive therapy has been reported to ease the pain around these tissues. Additionally, by improving the pliability of tissue around a scar, it can be made less painful.

As a result, massage gun therapy is not only recommended for sports injuries, but for post-surgery scar tissue treatment as well.

PRACTICAL PERCUSSION THERAPY BENEFITS

Apart from the health benefits of massage gun therapy, there are practical reasons why you may want to own one of these devices.

Some of them are:

You can use a massage gun at home for self-care. Sometimes leaving home for a massage can be a hassle especially when you are not feeling like it or are simply tired. Just rev on your massage gun and get to work on your muscles.

You can use them on your family or loved one.

Have a massage on the go. You can carry a massage gun with you anywhere.

You get direct feedback when massaging yourself. You get to learn about your body as your self-massage. This is highly recommended if you want to achieve a healthy life.

WHAT ARE THE POTENTIAL CONS OF MASSAGE GUN THERAPY?

OK, so we just discussed some key massage gun benefits, but what about the cons of massage gun therapy?

There are downsides to massage guns, including the risk of aggravating injuries or other chronic injuries. This risk is increased if the individual is using the massage gun incorrectly. These risks can be remedied through training on the proper use of massage guns.

Here are some cons of massage guns you should be aware of:

Incorrect use

You'll notice that we have insisted on knowing what you are doing with a massage gun. A massage gun is a tool, and that means it's only as good as the user. You run the risk of injuring yourself or not getting the desired results. We will discuss proper usage later. Also, don't forget to read the instructional manual on how to use the device. Always stay on areas of soft tissue. When the head of the gun start to bounce across the surface of your body, it is likely on a bony prominence.

THE RISK OF AGGRAVATING INJURY OR OTHER CHRONIC CONDITIONS

Apart from the injuries we have listed above, it's not recommended to use a percussion massager on injuries like sprains, broken bones, or large areas of swelling or bruising. Chronic pain conditions like hypertension, varicose veins, rheumatoid arthritis, and others could become worse if you use a massage gun. Find out from a doctor or therapist about your condition before using a massage gun.

MASSAGE GUNS CAN BE HEAVY AND BULKY

Some massage guns can be rather bulky and make using them a tough task. However, there are some that are compact and light. You also have the option of mini guns should the full-sized ones prove too heavy for you.

HIGH INITIAL PRICE POINT

This was a problem when these devices had just hit the market, and some of them are still quite expensive. However, we can confirm that with many devices now flooding the market, the prices have gone down quite significantly. We will discuss comparisons in a future article.

GENERAL PRECAUTIONS/THINGS TO KEEP IN MIND

Massage guns can cause pain. New onset of pain usually means you are applying too much pressure, or the speed is too high. Check that you are applying just the right pressure based on what area of the body you are massaging.

Avoid touching nerves. When you feel an electric shock-like pain, stop immediately.

Do not use a massage gun directly on bony areas, the spine, neck, fractures or wounds.

Only use them on muscles for complete assured safety. Otherwise consult an expert.

Do not use a massage gun on an area that has impaired sensation. If you feel you're not getting precise sensorial feedback, don't continue massaging that area. Chances are you are doing more damage than repair.

Do not use massage guns if you are on blood thinners (example: heparin and warfarin) prescription.

Seek medical advice first before using a massage gun if you have:

An inflammatory disorder

Warfarin and heparin prescription

Muscle strain, varicose veins, ligament sprain, high blood pressure, and conditions affecting blood vessels like thrombosis.

OTHER DEVICES

Thrive – Manufacturer of High-Quality Massagers and Hair Clippers since over 80 years.

Thrive 717W Massagers has 2 Massage Speed, 4 Exchangeable Attachments, Can be used with or without heat and a very powerful motor.

717W Powerful Handy Massager can be used on varying parts of the body such as –

Chest Massager

Shoulder Massager

Neck Massager

Back Massager

Abdomen Massager

Tummy Tucks

Legs Massager

Arms Massager

Feet Massager

Benefits of Using Thrive Massager (G-5)

Strong and Irregular Body Massaging function with electric heating function

Provide massage in large range of body areas due to large surface

Draining Effect on the body through heat

Pain Relief and Metabolism increase through Heat Function

Light Weight and Easy Handling

2 Massage Speeds and can be used with or without heating function

4 Exchangeable Massage Attachments

Made in Japan

15

MASSAGE MATS

Massage mats can be good for you. It can help soothe tired back muscles with its heat function and loosen tightness and tension with the vibration massage. The heat helps to increase blood circulation while the vibrations work to ease the day's stresses away. Aside from relaxation and increased blood flow, massage mats can also help restore muscle flexibility with stretching and correct poor posture.

WHAT ARE MASSAGE MATS ANYWAYS?

Massage mats are mats or pads made out of foam (or similar material) that provides a massage or acupressure relief as you lay on it.

They help with back pain and relaxation.

Some are electric and have heating options while others do not.

Some manufacturers call their product a massage mattress, but whether they call it a mat, a pad or mattress, we will call it a mat for the purposes of this article.

Massage mats can be placed on beds, sofas, or the floor.

The floor is usually the best option though, but as long as the surface is level and you can comfortably lay down, a massage mat can be used on it.

Some massage therapists use a massage mat on their tables for its heating option as they find it makes their client-patients relax more easily.

What Are The Benefits Of Using A Massage Mat?

Massage brings a multitude of benefits like relaxation, stress relief, and pain relief.

Massage mats specifically provide the following benefits:

1. Helps to decompress after a long day. A half-hour session at the end of the day or before bedtime helps the body relax and sleep better. A more relaxed body lowers stress levels and hormones in your body. Lower stress levels help your body recover quickly and repair itself during sleep.
2. The heat increases blood flow. Increased circulation helps to loosen your muscles. Increased circulation also makes your muscles less sore and help heal any microtears.
3. The right pressure on the body's acupoints helps to restore not just blood flow but also lymph flow. Lymph drainage flushes the body's lymph fluid and other impurities out of the body. This not only keeps you healthier but also energized when you wake up the next morning.
4. The vibration paired with the heat will bring relief to muscle soreness as well as break muscle adhesions and tightness in your back, shoulders, hips, and thighs. Treatments at the end of the day prevent the stress and injuries from building up.

Something To Be Aware Of

Massage mats are only for your backside.

It can't massage the side or front of your body.

So keep this in mind.

Typical Features

Not all massage mats are the same and have the same features.

With that in mind here are some of the more common features...

Foam cushion. Electric massage mats are cushioned making it look similar to a quilted duvet. The foam used varies, but some of the higher-priced mats are made out of orthopedic cushions or memory foam. When you factor all the materials that make up a massage pad you'll find that most weigh between 4-10 pounds.

Fabric covers. A very common cover is a polyester fabric that is completely washable. Some are plush, which makes it really comfortable to lay on. Another fabric commonly used is a sturdier fabric similar to canvas. Some covers aren't removable or washable but can be cleaned with a damp cloth or a disinfecting wipe (similar to what you use on a yoga mat).

Pro tip: If you want you could place a sheet or a towel over the mat during use to keep the fabric cleaner.

Built-in pillow and neck support. Massage mats are quilted like a duvet with some having a fuller headrest to cradle the head and neck. The pillows don't always have mechanisms or vibrating parts. Its primary function is to offer support for the head and neck and keep it aligned with the spine. There are some models that have a vibrating function or massaging nodes where the neck meets the shoulder to knead away stress.

Massage nodes. Some models are covered in plastic nodes with multiple pressure points that correspond to the acupoints in the body. Others may have nodes that move to massage away the tension and knots in your back and neck.

Heat. Some massage pads have a heat function to help relax the muscles. Most models just have an option to turn them on or off but no option to target certain areas of the body. The mechanism and technology for massage mats aren't as advanced as those found in massage chairs. The limited heat function keeps the costs down and the units more affordable.

Vibration. Due to the thin width of massage mattresses, adding shiatsu massage nodes cannot be done throughout the entire length of the mat. Vibration massage mechanisms are added instead. Different vibration intensities are usually an option. Some mats have shiatsu nodes in the pillow for the neck and shoulders.

Remote Control. In the remote control, you will usually have the following options: power, vibration, intensity levels, and heat. Some may include pre-programmed modes and settings and a selector to choose the areas where you want the massage (upper or lower back, thighs, or legs).

Carrying straps. Most mats are designed to fold for easy storage. Straps help to secure and carry it around like a duffel bag.

Are Massage Mats Safe?

Yes, they're quite safe to use.

Most models have an auto-shutoff function or preset timers so even if you fall asleep in the middle of the massage, you don't have to worry that you'll hurt yourself with an extended massage session or burn the house down.

Safe For Pregnant Women?

General massage is safe for pregnant women in their 2nd and 3rd trimesters but a massage in the first 12 weeks of pregnancy increases the risks of miscarriage.

However, we do not recommend you use a massage mat while pregnant.

The safest massage position for a pregnant woman is on her side.

This isn't possible with a massage mat and the vibrations may not be good for the baby and may trigger contractions.

Discuss your massage alternatives with your doctor if you feel that prenatal massage would be helpful in easing your pregnancy discomfort.

Good For Children?

Massage mats should not be used on children because it's not built for their bodies nor safe.

If you want to give your child a massage (kids can have stress too), stick with traditional touch therapy where your hands will be able to manipulate little limbs and adjust pressure as their body needs.

Thickness Of Massage Pads

The electric mats have a thickness between 1 to 5 inches depending on the brand.

There is foam padding to cover the massage mechanism inside the mat.

The massaging feel like flat pieces of plastic saucers when you lay on it.

It's barely noticeable, but may be uncomfortable for some when you're lying on it for long periods.

Conclusion

Massage mats are relaxing and effective for helping relieve tension throughout the body.

The mats with vibration and heat are really soothing.

The acupressure mats are really effective for reducing tension, and would likely benefit those with sciatica and neck pain.

Unfortunately, we haven't been able to find a good massage mat that has shiatsu nodes. They tend to break down easily and be quite expensive.

If you want something that has massage nodes that rotate, then we recommend trying a neck and shoulder massager or massage chair/pad.

Massage mats are quick fixes for some nagging pain and soreness you want to spot treat before it gets any worse. It works as a relaxation tool when you want to take the stress and tension away at the end of the day.

BIBLIOGRAPHY

JOURNALS

https://www.jocms.org/index.php/jcms/article/view/774

https://www.ncbi.nlm.nih.gov/pmc/articles/PMC4440196/

https://pubmed.ncbi.nlm.nih.gov/29548300/

BLOG

https://blog.phschiropractic.com/blog/the-3-types-of-whole-body-vibration

http://blog.myneurogym.com/study-finds-a-connections-between-the-universe-and-the-human-brainl

WEBSITES

Bedsores (pressure ulcers) - Symptoms and causes - Mayo Clinic

http://www.dr-randoll-institut.de/en/so-wirkt-die-matrix-rhythmus-therapie-marhythe/

https://www.mdpi.com/2411-5142/2/2/17

https://www.healthline.com/health/vibration-therapy

https://en.m.wikipedia.org/wiki/Matter_wave

https://www.practicalpainmanagement.com/treatments/rehabilitation/whole-body-vibration-potential-benefits-management-pain-physical-function#:~:text=Whole%20body%20vibration%20(WBV)%20is,mechanics%2C%20and%20quality%20of%20life.

Journal of Foot and Ankle Surgery (Asia Pacific) (jfasap.com)

EBSCOhost | 155401541 | Effect of matrix rhythm therapy in diabetic foot ulcer healing: A case report.

Application of matrix rhythm therapy (marythe©) for the treatment of decubitus ulcer in cancer Huddar V, Pattanshetty R - Indian J Phys Ther Res (ijptr.org)

Effect of Matrix Rhythm Therapy on Chronic Vein Dysfunction Deep Foot Ulcer: A Case Report (semanticscholar.org)

https://www.arktherapeutic.com/

https://mindbodypal.com/are-massage-mats-any-good/

CATALOGUE

Catalogue of Pro Vib (vibration platform)

BOOKLET

Concept of matrix rhythm therapy by Dr U Randoll Munich Germany.

NOTES FOR THE READERS

www.ingramcontent.com/pod-product-compliance
Lightning Source LLC
LaVergne TN
LVHW021159160826
845679LV00024B/2171

* 9 7 9 8 8 9 6 3 2 7 8 9 9 *